D1531217

POSTURE MAKEOVER

✳ ✳ ✳

The Secret to Looking Great, Feeling Confident and Living Pain Free

✳ ✳ ✳

by
Michelle Joyce

Posture Posse Press

Copyright © 2017 by Michelle Joyce.

All rights reserved.

Published by Posture Posse Press. Eugene, Oregon, USA

Cover art by Puk Fenneman.

978-0-9915148-4-7 paperback
978-0-9915148-9-2 ebook

Library of Congress Control Number: 2017949793

First Edition

Visit the author's website
www.posturemakeover.com

CONTENTS

✳ ✳ ✳

Whenever you see this icon, you can watch an accompanying video demonstration at

www.posturemakeover.com

Go to the "Book Club" tab and use the password

Postur3

for Steve,
my backbone

PREFACE

You can buy any number of gadgets and gizmos that promise to help you improve your posture. From designer office chairs and straps that hold your shoulders in place, to high-tech gadgets that buzz when you slump.

Here's the problem: none of these expensive toys actually work. Ergonomic chairs are of no use if you still slump while using them. Straps that pull your shoulders into place only create a downward spiral of dependency and muscle atrophy. And if your phone buzzes every time you slump, you're just finding out that you slump a lot, without ever learning how to break the habit.

But don't despair. Changing your posture is easier than you think. And you don't need to buy a bunch of stuff to help you do it. This book contains everything you need to know to get started on your journey to better posture. It's surprisingly simple.

First, you'll need to forget everything you've ever been told about "good" posture. The old chest-out-chin-up position is the opposite of what we're going for. Rather, we're making sustainable, life-long changes. And the good news is that it's not about willpower and strength. It's about relaxation and letting go.

Once you get the hang of it, you'll find that healthy posture is addictive. You'll notice some of the positive effects right away, and over time you'll notice many more. You'll look better and feel better. You'll have more energy and less muscle tension.

Before you start to worry that you can't do it, let me tell you a secret: your body already knows what to do. Healthy posture is natural, and chances are that you had beautiful posture when you were a small child. It's already familiar to your body, and the techniques in this book are simply ways to help reawaken the memory within.

I've helped many people change their posture, and they always react the same way, "Ah, that feels so much better." My goal is to get you to that place as soon as possible.

It took me a long time to learn the secrets to healthy posture, mainly because nothing like this book existed back when I started looking for answers. I had to dig deep for every nugget of information that I found, and figure out how the

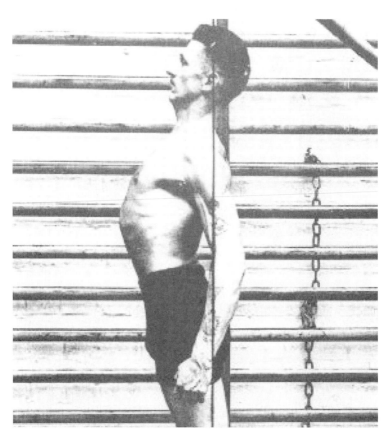

This old WWI recruitment poster is NOT an example of good posture.

whole posture puzzle fit together, borrowing concepts from modern medical journals and obscure books that had been out of print for more than a hundred years.

I uncovered buried wisdom in surprising places, and compiled all of it here. And I drew on my training as a Marriage and Family Therapist to expose the psychological and social barriers to breaking unhealthy posture habits. I wanted to make sure that this book addressed the whole person, not just a few body parts.

When I started my search, I would have given just about anything for a simple, step-by-step guide that explained exactly what I needed to do to change my posture. But that book never existed...until now.

We begin in Chapter 1 with the story of how my crippling back problems sent me on a mission to find the secrets of healthy posture and free my body from chronic pain.

You'll take the important first step on your own posture journey in Chapter 2, by making sure you start your posture makeover with the right mental attitude to set yourself up for success.

In Chapter 3, you'll learn the fundamental techniques that will allow you to retrain your body to sit effortlessly and dissolve the tension in your neck and shoulders that's holding you back from achieving better posture.

You'll put those foundational skills into action in Chapter 4, as you learn how to bend, walk and move with your new body. The straightforward instructions show you exactly how to stay in balance while you're on the go, whether you're cleaning up after a messy toddler, or out for an evening stroll.

We all need good posture role models, and you'll find plenty of them in next few chapters. We explore the mystery of why people from poor, rural cultures seem to experience so much less back pain than pampered office workers in Westernized countries in Chapter 5. And find out why your baby probably has better posture than you in Chapter 6.

You'll get my top ergonomic tips and tricks for avoiding common posture pitfalls in Chapter 7. These no-nonsense hacks will help you maintain great posture in any situation, whether you're stuck in rush hour traffic, or binge watching your favorite show on the family couch.

In Chapter 8, we delve into the science behind how healthy posture sends social signals that can make you appear sexier, skinnier and more successful.

I've also included several posture-improving stretches and exercises in Chapter 9, so you can mix it up and keep making progress at your own pace.

Finally, in a special bonus section, we'll rediscover a forgotten chapter in American history when posture was a hot button political topic, including the strange but true story of how naked photos of future presidents, Oscar-winning actresses and supreme court justices ended up in the archives of America's most elite universities – all in the name of posture.

Once you get started, there's no wrong way to use this book. You can read it all in one sitting, or work through it slowly, mastering each skill before moving on.

The fact that you've picked up this book means that you've already started to rewire your brain. From now on, it'll be difficult to see someone hunched over their phone without feeling the urge to reset your own posture. The seed has already been planted.

CONFESSIONS OF A POSTURE FANATIC

When I tell people that I'm a posture teacher, they always react the same way. First, they snap to attention like a military cadet, chest out and chin up. Then they confess that their posture is usually terrible. Sometimes they say that they're trying to get better, but mostly they sheepishly describe themselves as "lazy" or "bad."

A lot of people have told me that they're making an effort to improve their posture. One woman said that her whole workplace was on the posture bandwagon. One of her co-workers went so far as to set an alarm that would go off every 10 minutes to remind everyone to sit up straight. Every time the alarm rang, they'd all sit up straight as straight can be. But inevitably, they'd slowly slump back down to their original position until the alarm rang again. While their intentions were good, they never made any real progress towards changing their habits.

Simply telling yourself to "sit up straight" doesn't solve the problem. If anything, it perpetuates a cycle of discomfort and frustration that ultimately leads to giving up. We end up telling ourselves that good posture is too difficult and that we aren't disciplined enough. We give up on the possibility of change and resign ourselves to a lifetime of slouching, never realizing what we're missing.

I used to think that way too. I still remember sitting at my desk, pinching my shoulder blades together and puffing out my chest, shaking from muscle fatigue, feeling proud that I was doing something healthy. And when I sunk back into a slump, rolling back into my chair, I felt a guilty pleasure. It seemed so much more comfortable to collapse downward and let myself finally relax.

A Turning Point

I probably would have continued down that path if my back pain hadn't gotten so bad. I've been physically active my whole life, and I figured that back pain was the price I had to pay. As a teen, I was a nationally ranked competitor in horseback gymnastics (a sport called vaulting), and had fallen off running horses more times than I could count. I

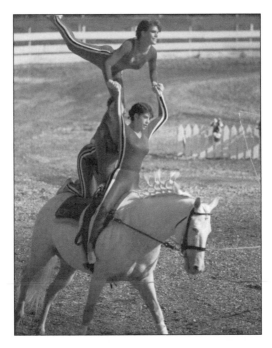

As an active teen I'd always assumed that back pain would be in my future. (That's me on the top!)

still remember joking with my teammates that we were all going to be in a lot of pain when we got old. And I was right!

Even as a kid, I'd assumed that pain was a natural part of aging, so I wasn't surprised when my occasional back pain started getting dramatically worse in my twenties. Around that time I'd become a competitive dancer, using every free moment to teach dance classes and prepare for the next dance competition.

Dancing was an obsession, until the doctor told me to rest my aching back after an MRI revealed that I had several herniated discs. I took months off to heal, but to my horror, the pain just got worse.

I started getting constant massages, acupuncture treatments, cortisone shots, chiropractic adjustments and I went to yoga classes. I can't even begin to imagine how much money I wasted trying to feel better. Nothing helped.

Dancing Through The Pain

Once I realized that resting my back didn't seem to help at all, I decided to stubbornly pursue my dance career. Then, I started getting invitations to perform and teach all over the world, so I quit my day job as a social worker and danced full-time. It was an absolute dream come true, or it would have been if I wasn't constantly worried that my body would suddenly give out, and that my newfound career would come to a humiliating end.

I remember getting off a plane in Tokyo, where I was about to teach a series of sold-out workshops, worrying that I might collapse to the ground at any moment. After sitting on the plane for so long, my back was worse than it had ever been. It didn't make any sense to me, since my back felt okay before I got on the flight. I now realize that the plane seat

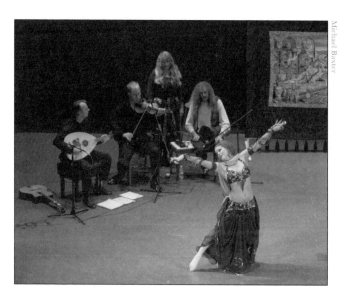

I still remember wincing in pain during this dance performance.

was pushing me into a slumped position, irritating my temperamental back.

Hiding the pain was exhausting, and I was constantly worried that no one would hire me if they knew the truth.

Just When I Thought It Couldn't Get Any Worse

When I wasn't teaching or performing, I was sitting in front of my computer, building a company that sold dance DVDs. I spent hours upon hours slumping in front of the screen, working late into the night. I was under the impression that sitting rested my overworked back, but (you guessed it) the pain just got worse.

By the time I got pregnant in my thirties, back pain completely dominated my life. In late pregnancy, I'd often have severe muscle spasms while getting out of a chair, sometimes collapsing to the ground. I never hurt myself or my baby, but it scared the heck out of everyone else! Driving was the worst because I always felt a shot of hot, sharp pain the second I got out of the car.

When my daughter was born, the pain didn't ease up. I was constantly bending over to pick her up, put her in her crib, nurse her and carry her around. When she was a toddler, I'd often sit on the park bench instead of running around with her, just so I could rest my aching back.

I thought my future was set, that my body was trashed and that I'd never get out from under the shadow of back pain. It continued to flare up and calm down at unpredictable times, and I couldn't make rhyme or reason of the patterns. I felt helpless and depressed.

Ignorance is the Opposite of Bliss

I'd all but given up hope when I read about an obscure school of thought that had been developed by a French woman named Noel Perez. She closely studied the posture of people in tribal cultures, noticing that they didn't tend to slouch the way that Westerners do. The most intriguing part was that back pain rates were reported to be much lower in these regions. Changing your posture, she said, could cure your back. That was the beginning of my metamorphosis.

As a dancer and an athlete, I assumed that being in good shape meant that I had great posture. But it turns out that I had a lot of misconceptions about what healthy posture looked like, let alone how to achieve it. And that's the problem with practically everybody I've ever met: **We think healthy posture is one thing, but it's actually something totally different.**

I never imagined that healthy posture could be comfortable, and that one day I'd actually prefer it to slumping. And, most of all, I never thought that I'd be able to hold my healthy posture all day long.

I always thought of great posture as something you did for show, like at a job interview, but that behind closed doors you got to let yourself off the hook and finally relax. I was pleasantly surprised to find that healthy posture is all about relaxation. And that it's effortless once you get used to it.

Cracking The Code

Being aware of my posture was a great start, but I still had no idea how to change. I had to be taught exactly how to undo my old habits and replace them with new ones. I didn't need to simply be told to sit up straight. I needed to learn *how* to do it.

I embarked on a journey of studying everything I could get my hands on. I delved into reading about obscure and forgotten techniques, hoping to uncover the secret to sustainable, healthy posture. I tracked down dusty, old etiquette books from the 1840s, trying to find lost pearls of wisdom. I dug through the archives at Stanford University, reading studies on everything from herniated discs to the possible link between texting and depression. I became fascinated with an influential group called the American Posture League that was responsible for creating a comprehensive posture curriculum for school children at the dawn of the 20th century.

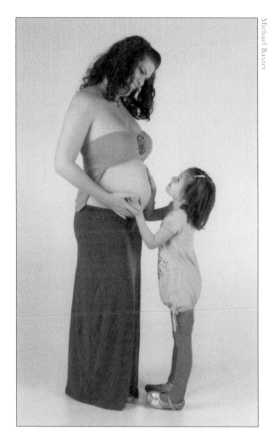

Changing my posture made my second pregnancy so much easier!

I talked to everyone I could find, studying the Alexander Technique and the Feldenkrais Method; analyzing the posture of rural, tribal peoples; and becoming certified in both Occupational Ergonomics and a form of assisted stretching therapy called Reposturing Dynamics. It's safe to say that I've become obsessed with posture.

The New Me

Improving my posture has changed my life. I no longer experience the back pain that I once had, which is reason enough to continue on this path. But I also feel better in other ways. My balance is better. I'm more confident and coordinated. I can sit comfortably for longer. I have more stamina. And I can literally breathe easier.

By no means is my posture always perfect, but my body no longer feels that collapsing downward is more comfortable. As a matter of fact, slouched posture now feels uncomfortable to me. I don't think of healthy posture as a chore. I prefer it. It feels good.

Today, I'm a posture coach and I have the awesome job of guiding others through the transformative process of changing their posture. I'm a complete believer in the power of posture to revolutionize the way you look and feel, as well as the way you're perceived by others.

Surprisingly, making the change itself was relatively easy. The most difficult part was actually finding the information and support that I needed. This is the book I wish I'd had.

ATTITUDE IS EVERYTHING

Congratulate yourself! No, seriously. Improving your posture is a healthy goal. As a culture, we seem to dread healthy goals, treating them like chores that will deprive us of all pleasure. Unfortunately, that attitude sabotages us before we even start.

Changing your posture is not like cutting your favorite food out of your diet. It's something that feels good. You shouldn't feel like you're suffering through the process of change, and I don't want you to let that kind of thinking take hold. It's counterproductive.

An attitude of positivity will lead you down the path to better posture, and as your posture improves, you'll feel even more positive. It's a virtuous cycle. It's not just touchy-feely rhetoric, there's scientific evidence that collapsed posture increases your level of cortisol – the stress hormone. By contrast, open, expansive posture can increase testosterone levels, which increase confidence. (By the way, testosterone isn't just a guy thing. Low testosterone in women can lead to a lack of energy, as well as anxiety and depression). In other words, healthy posture can actually change the chemical makeup of your brain, making you more confident and positive!

So in order to ensure you'll be able to achieve your goal, you need to agree to a few ground rules. Firstly, you're no longer allowed to say that you have "bad" posture. You don't. You're just seeking healthier posture. Bad posture isn't bad. It's unhealthy and painful. You aren't bad, and your body isn't bad either...let's just remove any judgment from the equation.

If You're Trying, You're Trying Too Hard

Secondly, you're no longer allowed to say that you're "trying" to change. You *are* changing. Saying that you're trying implies that it's difficult and you might fail. You will not fail. You're simply in the process of change. Maybe it's slow change for some, maybe it's fast change for others, but if you follow the advice in this book, it'll be impossible to keep from changing.

I once had a posture teacher who insisted that I eliminate the word "try" from my vocabulary altogether, no matter what I was talking about. She said that if I was trying to do something, I was trying too hard and wasting too much energy.

One day, I made the mistake of telling her that I was "trying" to get pregnant. As soon as I said it, I knew she'd remark on my language. I immediately felt frustrated because I was, in fact, trying to get pregnant and I wasn't sure what she wanted me to say instead. Not only was the process of trying to get pregnant emotionally charged, but now I had to listen to this woman tell me that I couldn't even say it right!

She smiled kindly and suggested that instead of saying I was "trying" to get pregnant, I start saying that I was "hoping" to. I took her advice and realized that it did feel better to say it her way. Saying that I was trying highlighted the disappointment and failure that I felt, but hoping was, well, hopeful! It was a small change, but it made a big difference in my attitude. And, in the end, I did get pregnant after years of "hoping."

It's A Process

If you find yourself feeling bad that your posture isn't perfect, then you've missed the lesson here. You must approach a posture makeover with the attitude of a student who is eager to learn. Have faith that your posture will change.

Instead of feeling like a failure by saying "my shoulders are rolled so far forward," say something like, "I'm in the process of moving my shoulders back." It might sound a little bit cheesy, but your mind and your body are closely connected. If your mind is sending signals of stress and frustration to your body, you'll never be able to relax into effortless, healthy posture. So much of changing your posture is about eliminating unnecessary stress and tension from the body, so you need to be sure that you aren't working against yourself.

Remember, your posture won't suddenly become "perfect" overnight (actually, I'm not so sure I believe that perfect posture exists). It's a process, and you'll need to change some deeply ingrained habits along the way. But the good news is that while some things might take a bit of getting used to, others will instantaneously feel right. Your body will start to crave more change, and one posture breakthrough will lead seamlessly to the next.

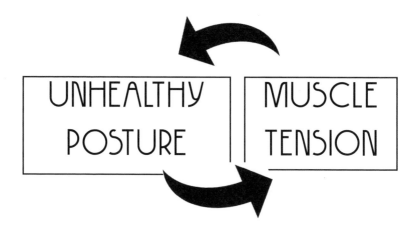

Step 1: Relax

We spend a lot of our lives sitting down, and all that sitting is changing our bodies for the worse. We spend so much time hunching in front of screens that our bodies are molding themselves into that position. Our heads and shoulders are perpetually pushed forward, causing muscle tension, which leads to even more unhealthy posture. This downward spiral of pain and tightness can only be broken once the muscles can finally begin to relax.

When you put yourself into a healthy position, your bones can do the job of holding you up, and your muscles can finally relax. Once your muscles start to let go, your body will naturally start gravitating toward a healthier position.

No Nagging Necessary!

One of my favorite clients was a teenage girl (I'll call her Ashley) with an extremely rounded upper back, slumping shoulders and a forward head. Like so many young people, she was experiencing chronic neck and back pain. Her mother had long suspected that her pain was related to her collapsed posture, so she was constantly telling her to sit up straight.

Part of the problem was that every time she heard her mother nagging, she immediately tensed up, feeling annoyed. Just thinking about her posture made her feel nervous and upset.

Another part of the problem was that she physically couldn't hold her shoulders back because her chest muscles had become so tight they were like rubber bands pulling her forward into a rounded position. Plus, her upper back muscles were extremely weak and stretched. This lack of muscle balance was at the root of her posture problem. She first needed to do some stretches and exercises to help give her both the strength and the flexibility to hold healthy posture.

Ashley's mother agreed to stop nagging. That gave Ashley the space to set her own goals, without feeling pushed into

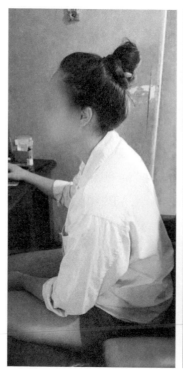
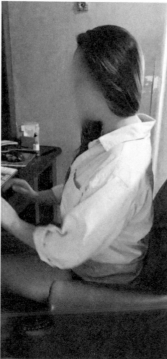

People who practice healthy habits in front of the computer are less likely to experience back pain. The posture on the left creates tension and tightness in the upper back, shoulders and neck.

it. She committed to changing her posture wholeheartedly, making her the ideal candidate for a dramatic change.

I prescribed some stretches to open her chest and arms, as well as some exercises to strengthen her upper back (I'll share those with you later). I helped her adjust her computer workstation, find a comfortable ergonomic position while driving, and gave her some tips about maintaining good posture while using her phone.

With just a tiny bit of coaching, Ashley's posture began to change. She's since gone away to college, but her mother tells me that her posture continues to improve and her back pain continues to fade.

It really can be that easy! As long as she keeps doing her stretches and remains mindful of her bad habits, Ashley's posture will continue to improve. And yours will too. All you need are a few pointers.

~ 3 ~

THE BIG THREE

The art of changing your posture is not so mysterious. You might be surprised at how incredibly straightforward it can be. Explaining the fundamentals of healthy posture can be done in just three bullet points. Ready?

1. Sit on your sweet spot.
2. Keep your head over your shoulders.
3. Open your heart.

That's it! I call them "The Big Three." As you start building these three healthy habits, your body will begin to change. Once you've mastered them, everything else will start to fall into place. Now let me explain what I mean.

Step #1: Sit On Your Sweet Spot

My biggest revelation came when I finally understood the importance of putting my weight on the correct part of my bottom while sitting down. When my weight was on this sweet spot, my entire body stacked up into beautiful posture without much effort at all. But when my weight was anywhere else, I was always a posture disaster!

I vaguely remembered hearing about my sitz bones in a yoga class, but before my posture obsession I didn't know exactly where they were, or why they were so crucial. Learning to sit on your sitz bones is the single most important thing you can do to set yourself up for successful posture.

Most people tuck their pelvis under when they sit down, putting all their weight back on their tailbone. It's such a common way to sit that many chairs are even designed to push us into that rounded posture. Resist! A chair with a firm seat and a supportive backrest will leave you feeling a thousand times better at the end of the day than an over-stuffed, bucket-shaped seat. Most people don't believe me at first, so you'll have to trust me on this one. Once you get a taste of how good it feels to have healthy posture, you just might find yourself with a new favorite chair.

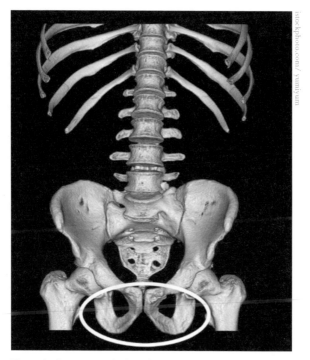

istockphoto.com/ yumiyum

Your sitz bones are designed to hold the weight of your entire body when you're sitting down.

The elusive sitz bones (aka the ischial tuaberosity) aren't always easy to find, but you can feel them pressing into the chair when you're on the right spot. Once they're properly anchored into a supportive chair, your spine and your entire body will naturally stack up straight all the way from your lower back, right up through your neck. If you aren't sitting directly on those sitz bones, you're doomed to fail, so let's make sure we get this step right.

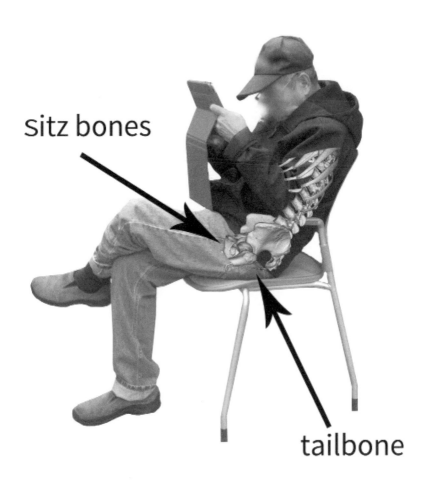

sitz bones

tailbone

When your weight is on your tailbone, it's impossible to sit up straight.

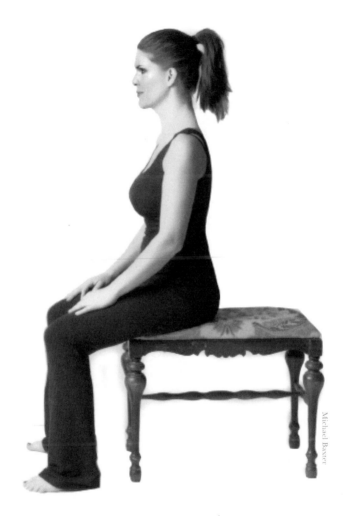

Sitting on your sweet spot is the key to healthy, relaxed posture.

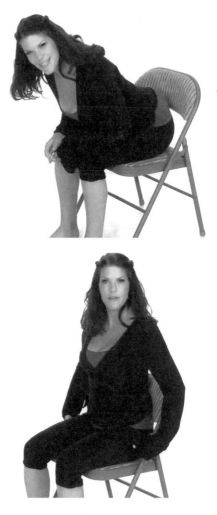

It's easy to find your sweet spot. Just lean forward, scoot your bottom back and sit up!

It's All About That Base

Luckily, finding the right position is easy. Just scoot your bottom to the very back of the seat, and bend forward so that your chest is close to your knees. When you sit up, your sitz bones will be firmly pressing into the seat. That's your sweet spot!

Go ahead and give it a try. Get yourself into the right position and give your body a moment to absorb how it feels. This will soon become an instinctive part of your muscle memory. Your body will naturally want to sit this way. But in the meantime, whenever you find yourself getting ready to sit down, pause for a beat, and remind yourself to set a strong foundation.

Never take that sweet spot for granted. Sometimes I find myself thinking I'm on my sweet spot, but my weight is actually slightly closer to my tailbone than it should be. At first I don't notice, because I feel like I'm sitting on a bone, but my back soon starts to fatigue, and my posture soon starts to sag. It's only when I reposition myself further forward that I realize my mistake. So don't be afraid to shift your weight around and experiment with subtle changes. Sometimes a tiny change can make a big difference.

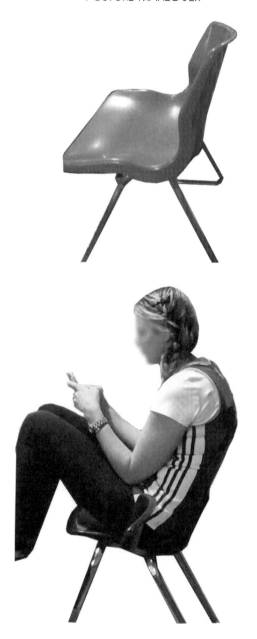

Bucket seats encourage you to sit on your tailbone.

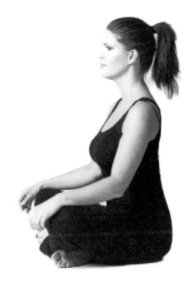

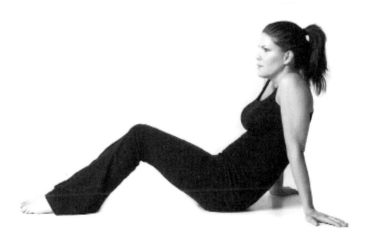

At first glance, you might think that the picture on the bottom shows a more relaxed position. Look again. The bottom position uses muscles in the arms, back and neck while the top position lets the bones carry the load, while the muscles relax.

I was sitting cross-legged on a blanket during an event at my daughter's preschool picnic when another mom said to me, "You must be exhausted. You've been sitting up so straight this whole time!" I got a kick out of that comment, because in truth, I was extremely comfortable and relaxed. It took very little energy to hold myself up, since my body was properly stacked up above my sweet spot. And, because I wasn't collapsing and squishing my internal organs, I suspect I was using less energy breathing and digesting too. Perhaps she was the one who was more likely to be exhausted!

Don't Cross Me

From a young age, women are taught to sit with their knees together, which is not a healthy habit. Squeezing your knees together all the time is taxing on your leg muscles and, since your leg muscles attach at the pelvis, it can create tension in your hips and lower back.

When I first started sitting with my knees a few inches apart, I immediately noticed that my lower back could finally relax. After years of suffering from chronic lower back pain and tension, it felt great to finally let that go.

All of the muscles in my hips were chronically tight, which pulled my pelvis into a forward (anterior) tilt. The muscles in the front of my hips (hip flexors) and groin (adductors) were cemented into place from years of holding them tight. Learning to relax those muscles was the first step to letting go of that chronic tension.

It's surprising how reluctant women are to let their legs completely relax when they sit. In certain outfits and in certain settings, I still squeeze my knees together, but it was difficult to overcome the habit, even while sitting at my desk with no one looking. It's not like I sit with my knees a foot or two apart (like every man I've ever been seated next to on a cramped airplane). I just separate them enough to be able to feel the muscles at the very top of my legs relax.

If you're used to those muscles being tight, it can be difficult to finally let them relax. It might help to visualize your knees gently lengthening away from your pelvis, creating more space in the hip socket.

I was also a chronic leg crosser. Almost every woman does it, but it creates that same kind of muscle tension, with the added disadvantage of pushing all your weight to one side. When your legs are crossed, your entire spine is out of alignment, which can cause tension all the way up through your neck. Learning to uncross your legs can provide relief to your whole body.

This can be a hard habit to break, so I've got a little cheat for you. Even though it's always better to have your feet flat on the floor, if you absolutely can't shake the urge to cross you legs you can cross your ankles instead (like the picture on the cover). That way you can keep your weight equally on both sitz bones, while satisfying the urge to cross your legs.

As a side note, if you Google "how to sit like a lady," you'll find that the crossed ankle position is supposed to be the height of feminine elegance and good etiquette. So, hey, if you're into that kind of thing, I guess that's a double win.

Step #2: Keep Your Head Over Your Shoulders

When my posture obsession first began, I was living smack in the middle of Silicon Valley, ground zero for tech workers. These industrious engineers and software programmers spend huge amounts of time hunching over their computers during long work hours, and it shows. Their extreme forward head posture makes them easy to spot. It's such a common problem that the media even invented a name for it – "iPosture" (aka the dreaded forward head).

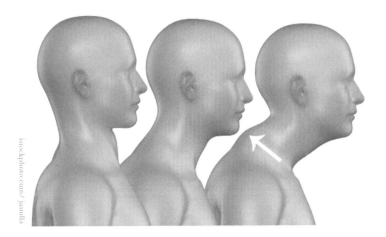

Forward head posture can cause chronic neck pain and a fatty neck hump.

Dump The Hump

I thought that Silicon Valley was the epicenter of the posture problem, since it's the center of the technology world. But then I moved to the sleepy college town of Eugene, Oregon. It's an outdoorsy community, the kind of place that seems to have a yoga studio and organic grocery store on every corner. I was expecting the general posture here to be healthier than in Silicon Valley, but I was shocked to find out that it's just as bad. In some ways it's even worse!

The University of Oregon is a magnet for young people from all over the world, most of them "digital natives" who've spent their entire lives in front of tiny screens.

I couldn't believe how many young college students had an extreme forward head, which is inevitably accompanied by a concave chest and slumping shoulders. It's sad to see young people in their prime setting themselves up for a life-time of neck and back pain!

Once you stick your head forward, even a little, your upper back muscles have to work overtime. The further forward your head goes, the more your muscles have to strain to keep it up. For every inch your head creeps forward, you add an additional 10 pounds of weight directly to your spine. So a 10-pound head can end up feeling more like it weighs 40 pounds, if it's just three inches forward.

The dreaded forward head typically has the added downside of being accompanied by a fatty neck hump at the top of your spine. That's because your body is laying down fat deposits in an effort to protect your neck from all that unnecessary strain. But don't worry, that fatty neck hump will shrink as your body adjusts to your new and improved posture. (I should note that a neck hump can also be a

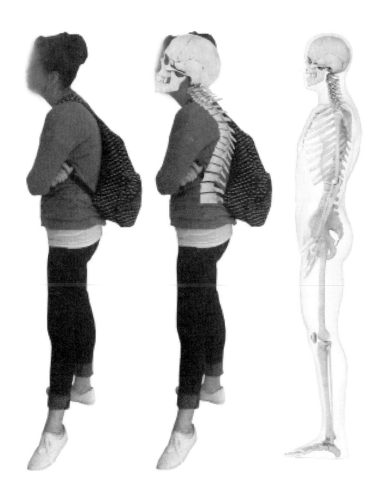

A forward head also comes with forward shoulders, a sunken chest and a rounded upper back.

symptom of other medical problems, so if you have one, it's worth mentioning to your doctor.)

Head and Shoulders Above of The Rest

When you push your big, heavy head forward, your body is suddenly much heavier in the front. To avoid falling forward, you must compensate by adding weight to the back. So then you round your upper back. But the chain reaction doesn't stop there.

A rounded upper back causes your shoulders to roll forward. And then the weight of your forward arms constantly pulls your shoulders forward even more. Then your back rounds more, your chest sinks further, and your head creeps further forward.

That's why it's so important to learn to recognize when you're holding your head forward. The most difficult part is noticing that you're doing it. Luckily, once you've identified the problem, fixing it is pretty straightforward.

It's All In Your Head

Start by gently lowering your chin. As you do this, you'll find that your neck will start to lengthen and the kink in the back

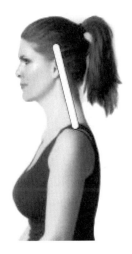 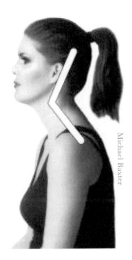

Michael Baxter

When your head is forward, there is a kink in the back of your neck.

of your neck will begin to disappear. Whenever that kink is there, you're working way harder than you need to in order to hold up your head. So the first step is to create length in the kinked area.

The next step is to get your neck vertical, rather than at a forward slant. The easiest way to do this is to give yourself a double chin! Or at least it'll feel that way. But don't worry, it doesn't look as strange as it feels. Plus, once your shoulder posture improves, the skin in the front of the neck will stretch tight again. So for now, please trust me on this one, go ahead and give yourself a double chin.

You may be using a lot of effort to hold your head in this position. That's because all of the muscles you use to pull your head forward have become stubbornly tight, not just in your neck, but all through your arms, chest and shoulders. We'll learn how to fix this in a minute.

For now, I'm only putting you in this position so that you understand where we're going with this. The chin tuck is an intermediate step that's meant to build muscle memory. Treat it as an exercise, not a position you're supposed to struggle to hold all day.

Your ultimate goal is to achieve this position through relaxation, even though it might not feel possible right now. Your head can literally balance on top of your neck with very little effort. The trick is to find that balancing point and relax into it. I like to focus on relaxing that spot right at the base of the skull, the place where the kink forms. It helps me to visualize the back of my whole neck relaxing and lengthening as my chin eases down.

Keeping your neck long and relaxed will take you a long way toward improving your posture. Once you've mastered this position while sitting still, start practicing nodding your head up and down without crunching your neck or jutting your head forward.

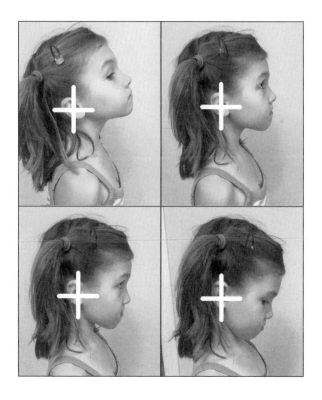

Practice keeping a long neck while you nod. Imagine that your ears are the fulcrum of the movement, staying still while your head rotates.

If you're struggling or frustrated, please back off from the position and focus only on relaxing. Simply lengthening your neck and letting your muscles relax is great progress by itself.

And remember, it's supposed to feel strange! The longer you've spent with your head forward, the more unnatural it'll feel to bring it back.

Step #3: Open Your Heart

People always think that when they come to me for posture coaching, I'm going to stand above them, make them puff out their chests, and criticize them when they can't hold that position for very long. I assure you, it's exactly the opposite. If they puff out their chest, I'll remind them not to.

I have no idea how puffing out the chest became mistaken for healthy posture, but almost everyone believes this posture myth. It's ridiculously uncomfortable and unnatural, but most people think it's great posture!

So please, fight the urge to puff out your chest. It's only putting an arch in your lower back that'll start to hurt before long. Instead, imagine opening your heart so that waves of relaxation radiate out from the center of your chest. As

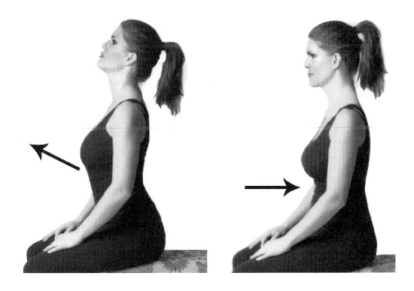

Most people think the photo on the left is great posture, but it's not. No one can hold that position for very long! The photo on the right is much more comfortable and sustainable.

you imagine your rib cage expanding in all directions, your upper back will become wider and your shoulders will relax away from each other.

The goal is to take up more space by expanding gently and effortlessly. I like to imagine that my ribs and shoulders are growing in the same way that a sponge expands when it gets wet.

To make sure you're not puffing out your chest, think about your lower ribs staying aligned with the rest of the rib cage. When your chest is puffed out, those lower ribs will stick out.

When your chest is tight, your shoulders will roll forward. It's possible to create the illusion that your shoulders are back if you puff out your chest, but you might find it difficult to get those shoulders back when your chest in a neutral position.

Roll With It

When your chest opens, your shoulders will start to move back. Instead of thinking about pinning my shoulders back (which creates tension), I think about putting my shoulder blades into position instead. Your shoulder blades should be flat against your rib cage and close to your spine.

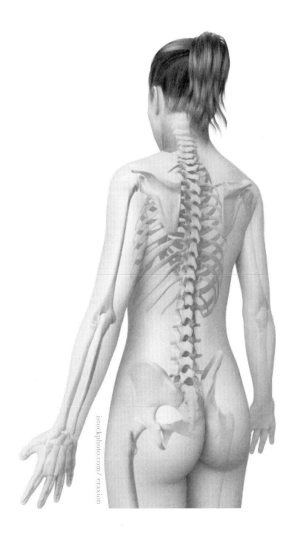

Ever noticed how anatomical pictures always show people with their palms facing forward? That's how your arms naturally hang if your shoulders are open.

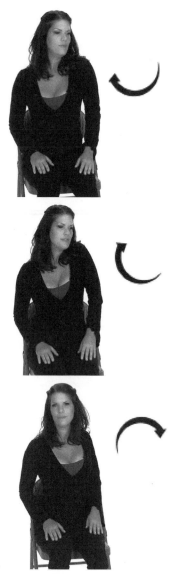

Shoulder rolls are a great way to get those shoulders back. One at a time, roll your shoulders forward, up, back then down (with extra emphasis on the back and down part). Then relax.

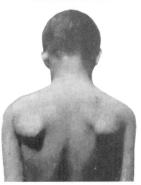

Don't wing it! Beware of "winged" shoulder blades that
stick out. Your upper back should be smooth and flat.

I also like to imagine that my shoulder blades are melting
into the back pockets of my jeans.

How do you get your shoulders into position without tensing
up? The shoulder roll! It's the perfect way to wake up your
upper back muscles and loosen up those tight shoulders.
Your body has been forced into that forward shoulder
posture from long hours of hunching over a computer,
which means you'll need to do frequent shoulder rolls in
order free your muscles from their old habits.

If you keep it up, you'll see results. Roll your shoulders
whenever and wherever you can: at every stoplight, before
checking your email, in the shower. Think of it as the latest
dance move – keep it loose and fun.

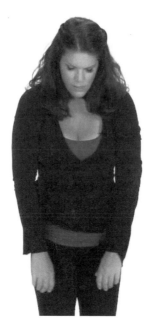

Looking at your hands is a great way to check your posture.
If your knuckles are forward, your chest is closed.

Stretch Goals

Let's take a moment to acknowledge the frustration that
you might be feeling at this point. If you've had unhealthy
posture for many years, your body has developed patterns
of tension and tightness that pull your shoulders forward,
even when you relax. Your tight chest muscles might be
yanking your shoulders out of position the second you stop
pulling them back.

This isn't actually as big of a problem as it seems. Muscles are flexible and will change with some consistent stretching and strength training. If you can dedicate just five minutes a day to posture stretches, your patterns will start to shift. Consistency is the key.

The problem is that good intentions can easily give way to busy schedules and old habits, and people start neglecting their stretches. If you ever feel too busy or tired, think of all the benefits you'll receive for your small investment of time and energy.

Stretching Will Save You!

If you need help motivating yourself to stretch, consider the results of a study out of Japan showing that a hunched forward position is a good predictor of how much care you will need as a senior. According to their research, those with long, straight spines will be less likely to need help dressing, bathing, eating and getting out of bed. So why not do your future self a favor and commit to doing these simple stretches?

For maximum success, I suggest doing your posture exercises at the same time every day as part of your regular routine. You can do it after you brush your teeth, while the

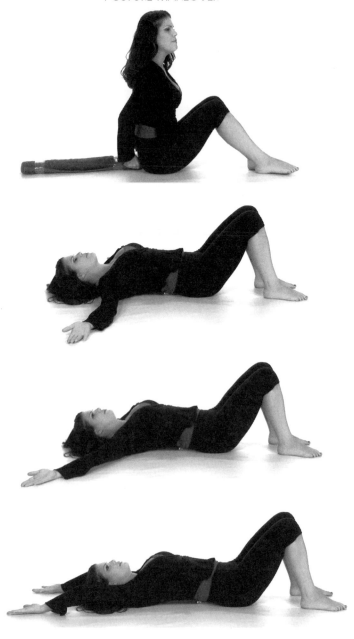

These gentle stretches open your tight chest muscles. I like to do them while watching TV at night, or in bed first thing in the morning.

baby naps, or during your lunch break. It doesn't matter when you do it. Just pick a time and commit to it.

Right now, I'm only going to ask you to do this simple chest opening series. Nothing more. Just this. And to make it even easier, it's a series of passive stretches, meaning that gravity does most of the work for you. (If you're feeling ready for more, there are many other stretches and exercises explained in the back of this book).

Rolled Towel Stretches

1. Roll up a towel and lie down with it directly underneath your spine (or roll two together for an even stronger stretch). You can wrap tape around the ends of the towel to keep it rolled up for next time.

2. Stretch your arms out into a "T" position, then take several deep breaths while focusing on releasing the tension from the front of the shoulders. Let your hands gently fall towards the floor with your palms up. If you want to deepen the stretch, you can hold some extra weight in your hands (like a couple of water bottles).

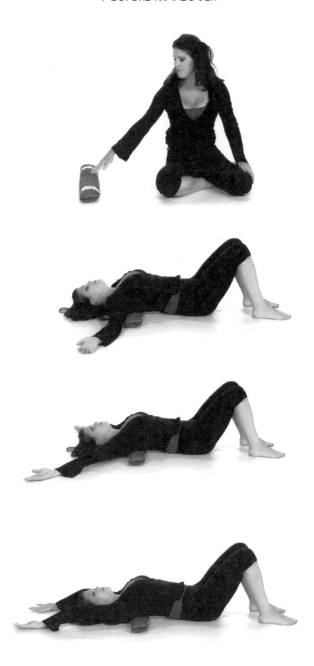

3. Repeat this sequence with your arms above your shoulders in a "Y" position. Then do it again with your hands straight above your head in the "I" position. Relax and let gravity do the work of opening up your shoulders.

4. Sit up and turn the towel sideways, so it is just under your shoulder blades, and repeat this series of stretches through the "T," "Y," and "I" positions.

The Next Step

As you continue stretching and working on "The Big Three," you'll absolutely start seeing changes in your body. And you'll find that feeling good is addictive.

Now that you know "The Big Three," it'll be much easier to navigate your way through those everyday moments that challenge your posture. These fundamentals can be applied not just when you're sitting, but also when you're on the move.

4

POSTURE IN MOTION

Once I threw out my back while gently bending down to put on my bedroom slippers. At the time, I was 23-years-old and in the best physical shape of my life, but the incident left me in bed for three days. I remember muttering to myself, "I'm getting old" as I sat in bed popping Vicodin and muscle relaxers (my doctor said that was the only "cure"). But what I should have said was, "My body is trying to tell me something."

It wasn't until years later that I started to rethink the way that I bend over. As a mom, it seems like I bend down a thousand times a day. I'm always lifting up my children, putting them into their car seats and picking up toys. I now know that every time I bend over, I'm making a choice. I can either

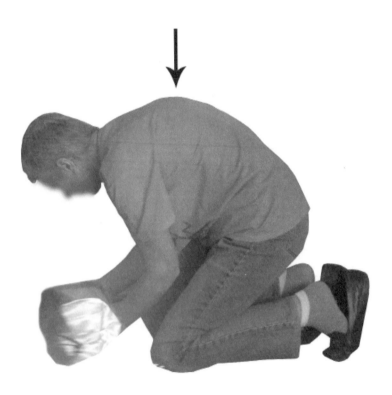

Ouch! That's gotta hurt. I'd be willing to bet that this poor guy has chronic pain at the apex of that curve.

compress my spine, causing unnecessary wear and tear on the spinal discs, or I can practice healthy posture.

I used to bend the same way that almost everybody else does: by rounding my spine. But now I bend from my hips, leaving my spine long and straight. It took a while to change my old habits, but I was finally able to do it when I slowed down and gave it some thought.

If you've been bending over the same way for a long time, your body is naturally going to try to do it the old way. **You need to stop and think about what you're about to do before you begin the movement.** I'm talking about literally stopping to think. If you start the movement without giving yourself time to make a conscious decision, your old habit will take over and you'll never change. In other words, tell yourself, "I'm going to bend over now. Don't let my spine round."

When you bend by rounding your back, you're squeezing the discs in your spine, causing a lot of wear and tear. This can contribute to the pain of bulging (herniated) discs and degenerative disc disease. I have both of these conditions, and I can tell you that learning to bend from my hips was one of the most important changes that I made to my posture.

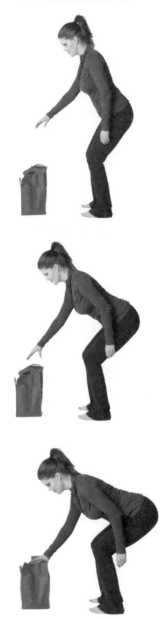

Bending from the hips takes some getting used to, but your back will thank you!

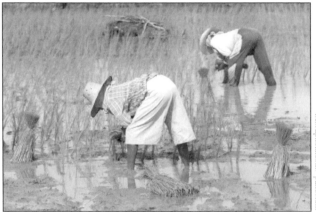

These farmers in Thailand bend from the hips and keep their backs long. This is a great hamstring stretch that you might want to try if you're going to be bending over for a while. I like to hang out like this when I'm picking up my son's Legos.

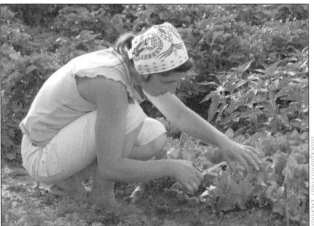

By contrast, this American farmer rounds her whole spine and rolls her shoulders forward to tend to her plants.

Bending From Your Hips

There are just a few things you need to think about as you bend. Visualize your tailbone moving up toward the ceiling, while your knees and hips bend. It'll take a while to get used to the feeling of sticking out your bottom, but rest assured, it doesn't look as strange as it feels!

A woman once told me about the first time that she used her new bending technique in public. She was in a restaurant when her scarf slipped from around her neck and fell to the floor, so she bent over to pick it up. When she stood back up, she half expected everyone to be looking at her butt because she felt self-conscious sticking it out like that. Of course, no one had noticed a thing!

So if you're feeling a little embarrassed about "hip hinging," you're probably doing it right! Don't worry, you'll get used to it.

At first it takes a lot of brain-power, but after some practice, it'll become a natural habit that you don't need to think about at all.

Walk The Walk

I had an epiphany when a good friend hosted a Japanese exchange student in her home. The student told us about the Posture Walking craze that had swept her country in the 1990s. A woman named Kimiko had opened walking schools all over Japan, becoming a famous figure with a cult following along the way.

I was curious how the process of walking, something we already know how to do, could become a craze in Japan. So I started taking a closer look at the way people walk, and I was surprised at what I saw.

Most people fall forward, slamming their feet down at the last minute in an apparent effort to stop themselves. Each step looks like it's about to end in a crash. It's an out of control, uncoordinated, unbalanced movement. Even many young people seem to almost limp along, modifying their walk to compensate for their forward shoulders and tight hips. And I noticed that most people swing their arms from side to side, instead of forward to back, a symptom of very tight shoulders.

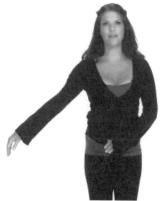

Many people swing their arms from side to side when they walk.

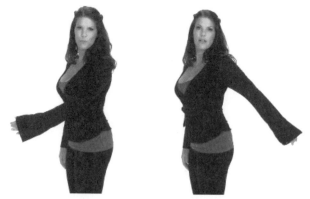

Try swinging your arms forward and back equally as you walk. It'll stretch your shoulders and tone your back.

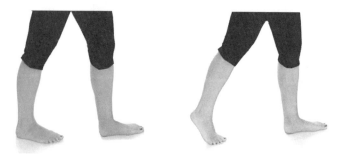

Give your hips a stretch by keeping your back heel on the ground for a split second longer. Then push through your foot to step forward.

Walk This Way

Making a few small tweaks to your walk can turn it from a culprit of unhealthy posture into a perfect form of exercise for posture correction. With each step you take, your shoulders and hips will open, and the weak, overstretched muscles in the back of your body will become toned and strong. It's surprisingly easy!

There are three main things to think about when changing your walk:

1. Swing your arms forward and back equally.
2. Plant your back heel on the ground with each step.
3. Roll through your back foot to propel your walk forward.

#1. Swing your arms forward and back equally. You might think that you already do this, but chances are that you swing your arms forward, but not back. When your arm swings back, it opens your shoulders and strengthens your upper back. The goal is to have equal-sized swings on either side. At first, you might want to try it as an over-exaggerated movement (like in the photo to the left), in order to imprint it in your muscle memory. With a little practice, it'll soon become an automatic habit.

#2. Plant your back heel on the ground with each step. As you do, straighten your back knee in order to feel a nice stretch through the front of your hip. I think about opening the back of my knee in order to put more pressure on my back heel. Resist the urge to lift your back heel until you absolutely need to.

#3. Roll through your foot to propel your walk forward. Think about rolling your weight through your foot, ending by pushing off with your toes. Be sure to wear flat, flexible shoes so that you can really feel the power of your foot to drive the movement. You'll feel how this engages the muscles all the way up the back of your leg right into your bottom. Forget booty toning exercises, all you need is a good walk!

A Walk a Day Keeps the Doctor Away

Now I understand the Japanese Posture Walking craze. Learning the secret to healthy walking is not just about comfort and fitness, it also makes you look confident and coordinated. A good walk makes a great first impression. Gliding into a room with comfort and ease sends an immediate message.

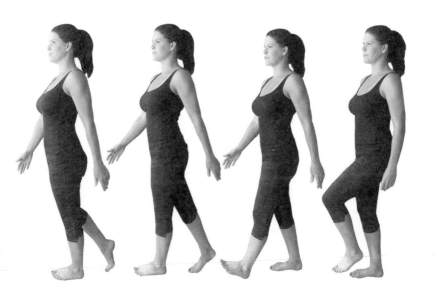

Practice staying upright while stretching your arms and legs
with each step.

Not only that, but walking for pleasure is the perfect antidote to sitting all day. Harvard University analyzed 47 studies that looked at the impact of sitting, and found that people who sat all day were at a higher risk of dying prematurely from a surprising range of diseases. Prolonged sitting has even been linked to higher rates of heart disease and diabetes!

Other studies have shown that working out regularly reduces these effects, especially if you exercise a little bit several times a day (as opposed to going to the gym for a burst of activity then sitting for the rest of the time).

Taking a few short walks throughout your day can improve your health so much more than you think. Once you get in the habit of taking walks, you'll come to appreciate the positive impact that the fresh air and endorphins have on your emotional well-being.

On the flipside, another study out of San Francisco State University found that walking with slumped posture could lead to depression and lack of energy. They also found that those feelings could be reversed simply by walking in an upright position. Amazingly, walking with good posture can help fight depression!

It's incredible that something as simple as taking a walk can have so many important benefits. If you can only spare three minutes to circle the parking lot, that's fine. It truly doesn't matter where you start, but it's important that you do.

Feeling Overwhelmed?

So far, I've suggested quite a few new habits and life modifications, and it probably feels like a tall order to incorporate them into your daily routine all at once. I know it's a lot to ask, especially since we don't usually have many good posture role models in our lives.

When learning something new, it's important to have people to emulate and learn from. You need good influences that show your body what to do. You may have heard of mirror neurons – they behave just the same if your doing a movement, or simply watching someone else do it. They help us learn to imitate what we see. So if you want to have healthy posture, you should spend time looking at people with healthy posture.

Worry not, I've left nothing to chance. The next two chapters are designed to show you plenty of examples of beautiful posture. I always feel inspired when looking at people who use their bodies to their fullest potential. I love being reminded of how incredibly graceful and strong our bodies are capable of being.

5

CULTURE SHOCK

In the late 1990s, scientists became aware that most studies about lower back pain were focused on high-income countries, which seemed like a major oversight. So a study was assembled to finally look at the other 85 percent of the world's population.

They didn't expect any surprises. Common sense dictated that people in industrialized countries would be in better condition. After all, we have access to quality healthcare and aren't subjected to the same sort of harsh conditions. Of course, they thought, an indigenous farmer who worked into old age would be more likely to suffer from back pain than a sheltered office worker in the West.

Boy, were they wrong. It turns out that affluent parts of the world consistently reported much higher rates of back pain. And while there were also back pain sufferers in the developing world, researchers found that they were mostly concentrated in urban areas. They even discovered some isolated, rural populations where chronic back pain was a relatively non-existent problem.

This head-scratcher sent researchers scrambling for possible explanations. They guessed that it might be because people in less industrialized countries get more exercise, are shorter, and have higher pain thresholds. But there's a simpler explanation. When you look at photos from these cultures, it's obvious that they hold themselves differently than we do. They're more in tune with their bodies, and they use them more efficiently. In other words, they have great posture!

They hold themselves that way because it is the most functional and healthy way to go through life. There's inspiring strength behind the elegance of their movement. It's not unusual to see women in Africa routinely carrying loads on their heads that total 70 percent of their body weight. And with healthy posture, they make this impressive feat look effortless.

In some pockets of the planet, whole populations naturally hold themselves with beautiful posture. They don't take posture classes and their mothers aren't nagging them to sit up straight. They just hold their backs long and straight without thinking about it. It's an ordinary, lifelong habit. But as industrialization sweeps through the world, populations like these are becoming harder and harder to find.

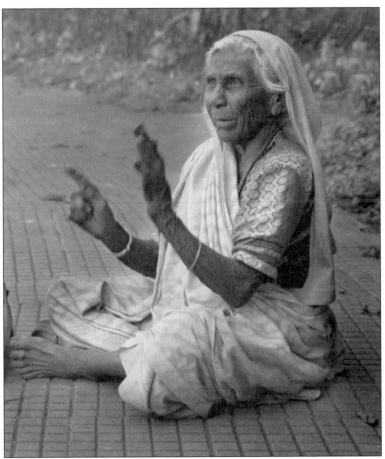

This elderly woman from India has beautiful posture.

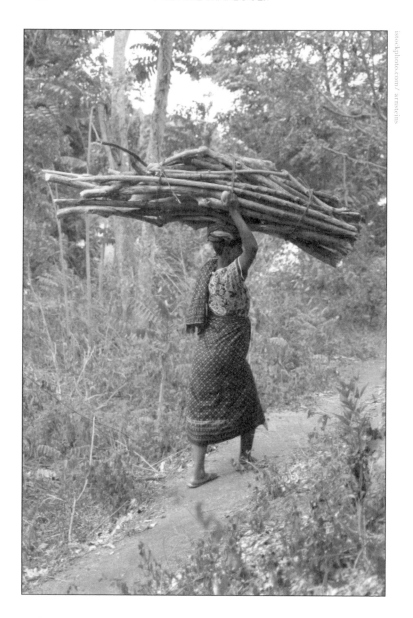

Despite that heavy load, her neck has a quality of length and relaxation. And look at that back heel pressing into the ground!

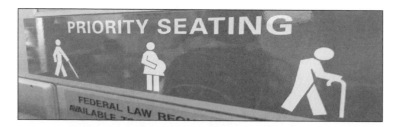

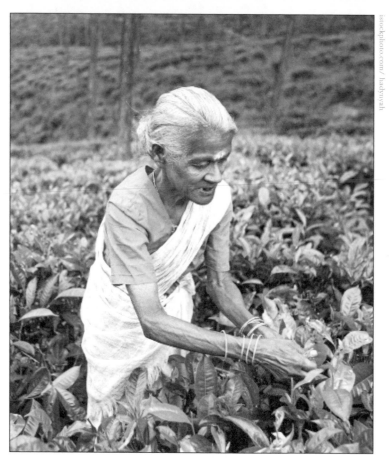

Top: This sign from a train in America portrays an elderly person with a hunched back and a forward head. The woman in the bottom photo shows no sign of hunching despite her advanced age. A lifetime of bending from the hips has served her well.

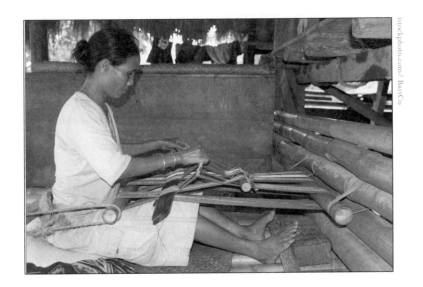

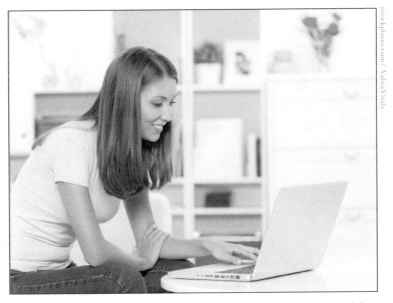

Though the Indonesian woman in the top photo may have a more labor-intensive lifestyle, the woman on the bottom is more likely to suffer from back pain.

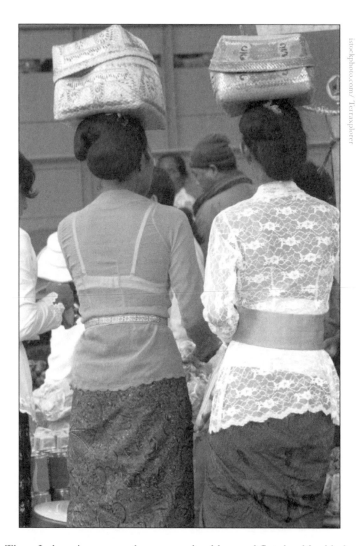

istockphoto.com/ Teraxplorer

These Indonesian women have open shoulders and flat shoulder blades.

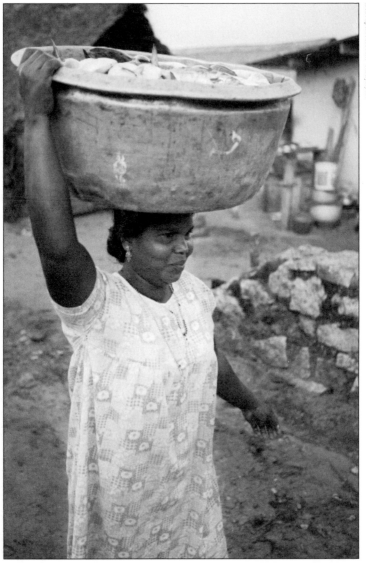

You can go to the gym as much as you'd like, but this kind of strength
comes from healthy posture.

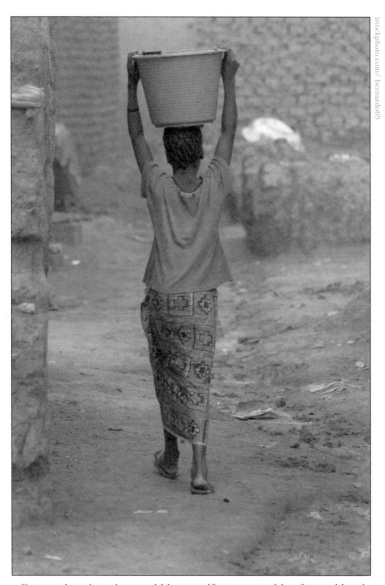

istockphoto.com/ bernard69

Can you imagine what would happen if someone with a forward head attempted this?

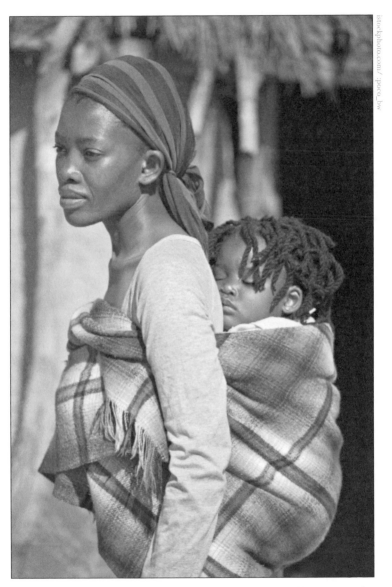

This mom carries her baby next to the strongest part of her core — her spine! Notice how her neck is long and her body is upright.

6

POSTURE MOMS

Your Toddler is a Genius!

Want more posture role models? If you have a toddler, you have a posture guru living in your own home! Babies have amazing posture. From the moment they learn to hold up their heads, they're constantly seeking the easiest and most efficient way of doing things. They have long, straight necks, so their heads can literally balance their heavy heads on top. It's effortless. Just look at any toddler, and you'll see what I mean.

The Three-Year Slouch

When my preschooler started slouching, I was very concerned. As a toddler she had pristine posture, but right around the three-year mark her long, straight sitting

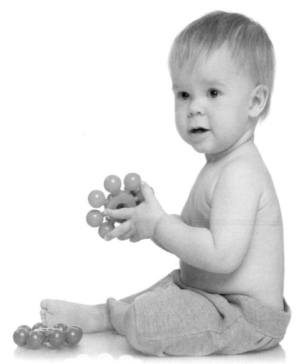

This little guy has found his sweet spot! He's balanced from top to bottom.

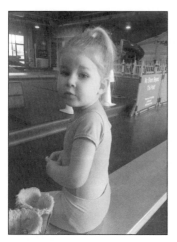 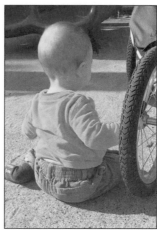

Toddlers usually have great posture. But around the age of three, their posture changes dramatically.

position morphed into a collapsed slump. As she spent more time at preschool and in front of screens, her posture got worse and worse.

When I started looking at the other children at her school, I noticed something that I couldn't believe had not occurred to me before. While her fellow three-year-olds had all adopted the same droopy slump, all of the younger children in the two-year-old class still had fantastic posture. What happened between the ages of two and three to cause such a shocking change?

Is it because they spend more time sitting in front of screens? Or because they're better able to balance and they no longer need to do things the easy way? Is it because of unsupportive furniture? Are they are trying to emulate the collapsed posture of the adults around them?

I thought I was about to embark on a long and difficult road getting my daughter back on track. I wondered if a three-year-old had enough self-awareness to make posture changes. But it turns out kids aren't all that attached to their posture habits.

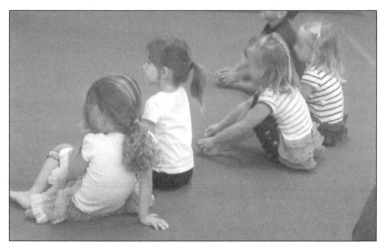

Can you guess which one is my daughter?

Your Preschooler is a Genius, Too!

I was surprised at just how easy it was to get her to revert back to the great posture she had as a toddler. Kids are eager to learn about their bodies, and as long as you make it a game, they're usually enthusiastic. My daughter was in a princess phase at the time, so I told her that slumping made an imaginary crown fall off her head. She would constantly ask if the crown was still on her head, and if she had healthy posture I would tell her, "Yes."

We even made up a game with Slumpyback Goblins, invisible creatures who pushed us into collapsed posture. We had great fun fighting them off when they tried to slump us down. We even turned this idea into a children's book called *Posture Posey and the Slumpyback Goblins*, and my daughter still takes great pride in being the real Posture Posey. So in a way, she feels like her healthy posture has earned her celebrity status. Just ask anyone who has ever visited our house and been forced to accept a copy of our book that has been carefully autographed with her best penmanship!

Don't get me wrong, it's still an ongoing battle to keep her from developing bad habits. But she knows that if she wants to play games on my phone, she's going to have to use healthy posture. That's the rule. When we're sitting at the dinner table, healthy posture is just part of having good table manners. Just like I remind her to say "please" and "thank you," I remind her to relax her shoulders and put her bottom in the chair properly.

Tiny Body, Tiny Chair

It's almost impossible for a small child to sit up straight on a couch. Their tiny bodies become engulfed in the sea of pillows and soft cushions, causing their backs to round in search of support. Their growing bodies need a firm chair that fits them properly.

Now, if I were to tell an adult that they couldn't sit on the couch anymore they'd rebel immediately! (Actually, we're going to have a heart to heart about your couch in the next chapter). But kids like having a special chair of their very own.

When my daughter was three, I bought her a little pink, plastic chair. It wasn't expensive or fancy. It was just a kid-sized, hard chair with a flat seat (not a bucket seat that dips down in the middle) and a simple backrest.

I told her that she was a big girl now, and that she was getting a very special new chair. Then, whenever she asked me if she could watch cartoons, I'd say, "sure, let's get your awesome new chair." In her mind, that chair became linked with her favorite shows. If she was slumping in her chair, I'd say, "let me make that more comfortable," while gently sliding her pelvis all the way back so she was sitting properly on her sitz bones.

I was consistent and enthusiastic, making sure I never scolded her when she slumped absentmindedly. I always framed it in terms of comfort. She knows that I want her to think about her posture because I love her and don't want her to get an achy back.

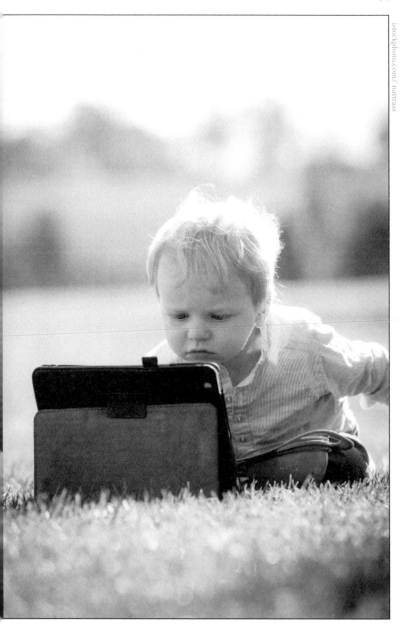

This screen is too low. See how it encourages this little guy to slouch?

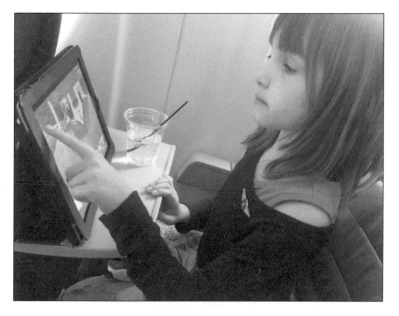

Long flight? Try placing your child's screen on the tray table to keep them from collapsing forward.

Muscle Memory Never Forgets

If they aren't taught any differently, most kids will start to slump. This was the case with my friend's daughter. She had the kind of droopy posture that's typical of a third grader, except for when she played the piano. When she sat down at the bench, she always sat with the most beautiful posture.

Anyone who's ever taken piano lessons knows that a good teacher will insist that you sit up straight before you even think about touching the keys. It might be hard at first, but most students adjust quickly. And before long, the habit becomes so ingrained that they find it hard to play the piano any other way.

That's the power of muscle memory. Your body automates certain movements that you do all the time in order to free up brain power for other tasks. That's why it can be so hard to break an old habit, because you are literally rewiring your brain! But that's also why it's so important to help children to develop good habits.

When it comes to screen time (that inescapable aspect of modern parenthood), try thinking about it the same way a piano teacher thinks about playing music – it's always better to do it with healthy posture. If you're consistent and supportive, the habit will develop. And it will last a lifetime.

iPosture

Like most parents, I let my kids play with my phone. But only if they promise to use healthy posture. This isn't as difficult

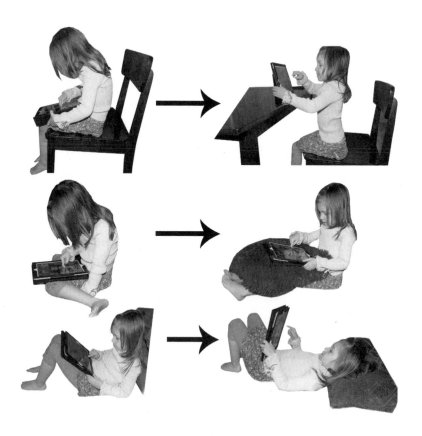

Small changes can make a big difference.

as it seems. Simply teaching your kids how to ergonomically hold these devices can save their posture down the line.

For example, at a table I'd ask my daughter to hold the phone upright on top of the table, rather than placing it flat in her lap. Just making that one simple change means she can comfortably watch the screen in front of her while keeping her head upright, instead of slumping down towards a screen in her lap.

If she's not at a table, I place a pillow in her lap and have her hold the device on top of that. Or, I suggest a reclined position where her back is flat.

As long as you remind your kids that you're helping their bodies to be more comfortable, they usually won't protest. In reality, they just want to get on with the business of playing with the iPad. They don't care if it's on a pillow or not!

If they start to protest, you can simply flex your parental muscle and tell them that they're only allowed to use it if they use healthy posture. That's the rule in our house. When my daughter asks if she can use the iPad, I say, "Sure, as long as you don't slump."

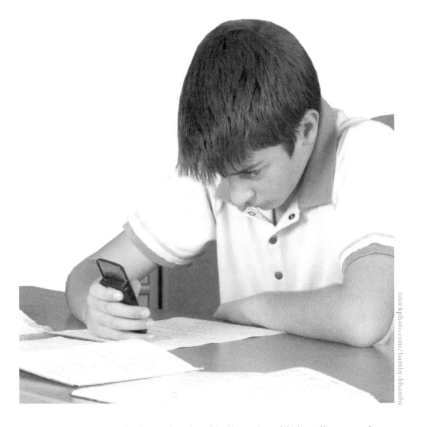

Childhood back pain is on the rise. I believe that this is a direct result of unhealthy screen time posture.

Whenever I notice that she's sitting up straight, I'm sure to tell her that she looks great. I tell her that I'm so proud and that she's doing a great job.

Watch My Back

I've asked my daughter to help me with my own posture, which is a bit of a mixed blessing! She loves loudly calling me out if my shoulders roll forward or my back rounds. To be honest, she can be a bit of a nag sometimes. But she feels like she's got an important job, and I do everything I can to treat it that way.

Whenever she says I'm slouching, I immediately change my position and thank her for the reminder. In turn, she never complains when I remind her about her posture. We treat posture reminders as little favors that we do for each other out of love.

I also treat her as my posture consultant. Sometimes, if she's slouching, I ask her if my own shoulders look rolled forward. It gets her thinking about shoulder position in general, and she'll usually unconsciously change her own posture. It's a sneaky way to get her to do a posture check without nagging.

Unfortunately, I had to rein her in a bit when she started publicly critiquing the posture of strangers! We had a few embarrassing moments for sure, but at least she was always quick to follow up her posture critique with a compliment. Such as saying, "You're slumpy, but I like your bushy beard," to the large man at the grocery store who was wearing a leather biker vest. At least he had a good sense of humor about it.

Children can be the most diligent of posture buddies because they love to be involved in things that matter to you. When changing your posture is something you do together, you'll see great results. If you have a good attitude about changing yours, they'll have a good attitude about changing theirs.

That Post-Baby Slump

Motherhood is murder on the back. You're always lifting heavy things and carrying them for long periods (sometimes for nine moths at a time!). And when you aren't doing that, you're bending over awkwardly to put your baby in the car or lift them over the side of the crib. It's a posture disaster.

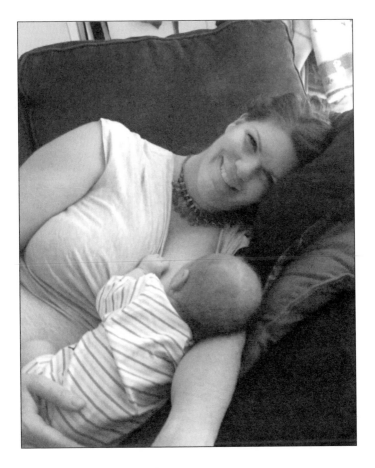

Bringing the baby to the breast, instead of the other way around, will spare you from neck and shoulder pain.

I started my posture obsession when my first child was a toddler. By the time I had my second baby, five years later, I was well practiced in the art of minding my posture. I remembered how much pain I'd been in, so I vowed to be hypervigilant about my posture the second time around.

And the difference was night and day. Even though I had muscle tension, it never hurt in that chronic, wincing way that I'd experienced before.

Hey You, Come Here!

I always made an effort to be "comfortable" while breastfeeding my first baby. I'd casually fling my leg over the arm rest of the couch, folding my torso around her tiny body. I spent hours and hours contorting myself and inflaming my back. But with my second baby, I took a whole new approach. I allowed my body to lengthen and relax while nursing. I sat in a firm chair with two pillows propped under my son's back. If two pillows didn't bring him up to my breast, I'd use three. I absolutely refused to bring the breast to the baby. I always brought the baby to the breast.

That tiny change completely transformed the way I felt. There was more freedom in my upper back, and feeding time became much more comfortable. I was able to completely relax my body and enjoy the time with my baby, instead of constantly shifting around in search of comfort.

Get Even

If anyone holds the world record for carrying a large amount of awkward stuff at once, I guarantee you that person is a mom. Even on my worst day, I can hold a baby, a bag of groceries, a dog on a leash and my purse while still stopping to open the mailbox.

It turns out that there's an art to carrying things. My mother sent me to a series of etiquette workshops when I was 12-years-old (kinda strange, I know). Among other things, they taught us how to "correctly" carry things. They said that we should always load everything onto the left arm so that the right arm was free in case we needed to open a door or something. It turns out that I'm lucky none of my etiquette lessons seemed to stick!

While it's nice to have a free hand, it's even nicer to have a balanced body. If you're always carrying things on one side, then you're making yourself lopsided. Whenever possible, evenly distribute the weight in both hands. Or, if you're only carrying one heavy thing (like a baby) it's important to avoid carrying it on the same side every time. Switch it up. Your body will thank you.

As long as you use common sense and avoid contorting your body, you'll be able to avoid a good deal of muscle pain. Of course, this advice isn't just limited to motherhood-related activities. It applies to everything that you do. But even the most posture-conscious person can fall into everyday posture traps. That's why the next chapter is all about resisting collapsed posture, even in the most difficult situations.

7

POSTURE TRAPS

Sometimes it seems like our whole modern world is designed to force us into the worst possible posture. I pondered this reality while sitting on an uncomfortable bench at an amusement park a few years ago. Someone had gone to a lot of effort to design a bench with a rounded bucket seat that made it impossible to keep from rolling back onto my tailbone. I'm sure it would have been cheaper and easier to build a traditional bench, with a horizontal seat and a vertical backrest, but this one was carefully crafted to push me back into a collapsed heap. That's what we've come to define as comfort.

We desperately need to build new memories in our bodies about what true comfort really feels like. Because I'd been training my body to crave healthy posture, that bench was the most uncomfortable thing imaginable. But I saw several families sitting on the same kinds of benches looking perfectly content. They were under the impression that they were comfortable, but in reality they were heavily taxing their bodies.

Don't Phone It In

I went to visit my husband one day when he was working at Stanford University. He'd warned me about the perils of driving on campus, but I thought he was probably exaggerating a bit. When I pulled onto campus, there were students everywhere, and almost all of them were looking down at their phones. At every intersection, hordes of pedestrians absentmindedly stepped out into the street, barely glancing up from their phones to double check that they weren't in the path of a speeding truck. Bicyclists swerved all over the street, only halfway paying attention to the busy environment around them. Many of them were riding with one-hand (or no hands), their faces staring down at their phones as they pumped away at the pedals.

While the driving situation was stressful, I was even more disturbed by the realization that many people can barely look up from their phones, even in potentially life threatening situations. And most of us hold our dang smartphones the same unhealthy way.

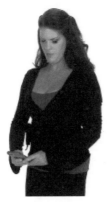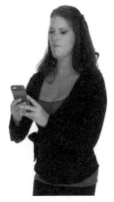

Take a moment to notice how you hold your phone. Does it feel better to hold it up higher?

Our posture is at its worst when we're looking at our phones. Most people hold them down low, below the chest, craning their heads forward, rounding their backs, and folding their whole upper body down toward the screen.

Next time you send a text, try lifting your phone just a few inches higher. It's not that much effort to bring your phone up closer to your face. And when you look down at the phone, be sure to lengthen your neck upward. Remember the lesson in Chapter 3 about using your ears as the fulcrum of the movement, letting your head pivot around them as you look down. You can also think about looking down with just your eyes, instead of your whole head.

You'll be amazed at how much this simple change will transform your posture! You'll instantly feel the difference.

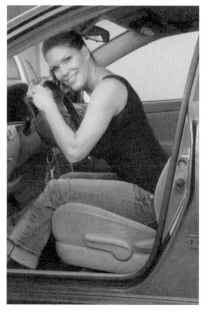

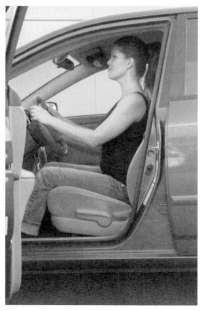

The bucket seats in cars make it difficult to sit on your sweet spot. Be sure to scoot back and sit on your sitz bones.

Don't Let Your Car Drive You

Have you ever been driving along, then felt the need to adjust your rearview mirror downward? That's not because your mirror has moved – you have.

A highway patrolman who spends his whole day behind the wheel recommends this next trick. He says that he doesn't adjust his rearview mirror while driving. Instead, he adjusts his body. As soon as he can see out his rear view mirror again, he knows that his body is right back where it needs to be.

In order to do this trick, it's important to take a moment to get yourself situated when you first climb into the driver's seat. Before turning the key, check your posture and adjust your mirror.

The car is a particularly problematic posture hot spot, because there's a bucket seat forcing your spine into a rounded position. Getting your bottom way back in the seat is important. Just like in a regular chair, you need to find the sweet spot where your sitz bones are firmly anchored in the seat. If you put a small pillow behind your lower back, it'll help support that healthy position.

The one and only good thing about car seats is the head-rest. At least it's easy to monitor your head position. Simply check to see if your head has crept forward by noticing how far away you are from the headrest.

Face It

I was recently at a doctor's office and the receptionist had a work setup that would be familiar to many people. She greeted clients at the counter as she faced forward in her chair, but her computer was positioned 90 degrees to her right. This "L" shaped setup meant that she was constantly twisting and contorting her body as she switched her attention from the counter to the computer.

It would have been much healthier for her to rotate her whole body, including her chair, but she got into the habit of twisting her spine instead. This kind of motion, day after day, can cause extreme back pain!

I catch myself doing this when I'm unloading the dishwash-er. Sometimes I absentmindedly pick up the dishes and twist my spine in order to put them in the cupboard, but I should be turning my whole body instead.

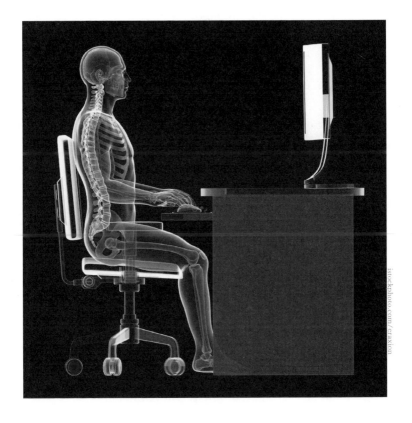

This is a nice ergonomic setup. His monitor is at eye level, his upper arms are vertical and his wrists are neutral. He's not twisting. He's close to the keyboard, and he's on his sitz bones. A shorter person would have to lower the monitor, raise the chair and add a footrest.

That repeated twisting puts an unnecessary strain on my body. When I remind myself to point my whole body toward the task at hand, I immediately recognize that it feels more comfortable and coordinated.

Make Your Office Ergonomic

I had to write a thesis in graduate school, which meant that I spent a lot of time in front of the computer. And, not coincidentally, I started experiencing a lot of pain in my right wrist and forearm. That's my mouse hand, and eventually the pain got so bad that I tried switching the mouse to my left side. That didn't work so well. So I bought an expensive, ergonomic mouse. That didn't work either.

When the pain started radiating up into my shoulder and neck, I finally went to a physical therapist. He told me that my computer setup wasn't ergonomic, and that making a few small changes would help relieve the pain (he also prescribed a few stretches and exercises).

Even though I had a keyboard tray at my work station, my mouse was up on the desk. The physical therapist suggested that I put the mouse down on the tray, as close to the keyboard as possible, and that I scoot my chair in closer. I was skeptical that this small change would put a dent in the pain

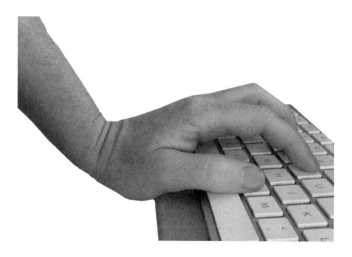

This keyboard is too low. Holding your wrist at an unnatural angle can cause chronic pain.

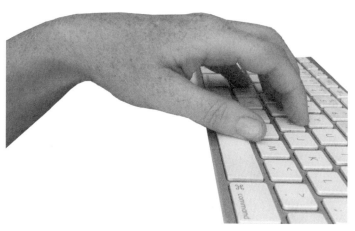

This keyboard is too high, and can also lead to chronic pain.

I was experiencing, but it really did! I haven't had the pain since. (I've since ditched the traditional mouse and use a tablet mouse instead).

I think that people feel intimidated by the idea of ergonomics, mostly because there are so many ergonomic products on the market. But having an ergonomic workspace isn't difficult or expensive. You just need to use common sense.

For example, you don't need to buy an expensive chair, just think about "The Big Three" while sitting on the chair that you have. You're better off adjusting a cheap chair than slumping in an expensive one.

Just remember, everything revolves around "The Big Three." My mouse injury would probably never have happened if I'd been in the habit of doing regular shoulder rolls and thinking about keeping my shoulder blades flat. When I reached all the way over the keyboard to use the mouse, I not only rolled my whole shoulder forward, but I also created sustained muscle tension in my arm. And that's all it takes to cause a painful injury. Especially if you do the same motion every single day.

Typing is terrible for your body. Remember how we learned that open shoulders cause your palms to face forward? Well, typing forces your hands to face the opposite direction, so you really have to be careful that you don't let your "back-ward" hands roll your shoulders forward.

When your hands and arms are already at an unnatural and vulnerable position as you type, it's extra important that your keyboard is at the correct height. It's in the right spot if your forearms are at a slight downward angle. Your wrists should be neutral (straight). If your keyboard is too high or too low, the repetitive motion of typing could lead to chronic pain.

Not sure where to put your monitor? "The Big Three" comes to the rescue again! When adjusting my monitor, I close my eyes and find my ideal neck position first. Then, after my neck is comfortable, I slowly open my eyes and see where my gaze naturally goes. That's where I position the center of my monitor. A low monitor will make you slump forward, while a high one will give you a neck kink.

Ouch My Couch!

If our great, great grandmothers were alive today, they'd gasp in horror at the furniture in our living rooms. In the 1880s, the "lounge" was introduced, and doctors issued public warnings about the harmful effects of sitting on such soft, unsupportive objects. They said that slouching on the

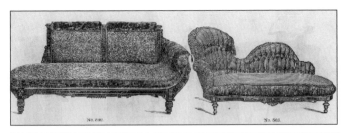

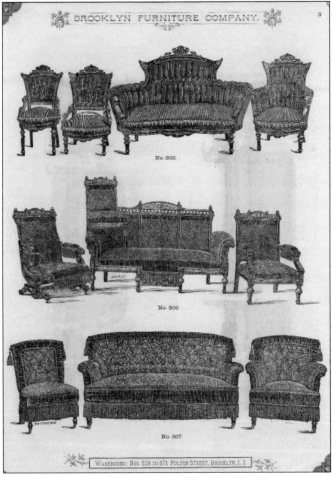

This furniture catalog from 1883 shows the trend toward softer chairs. Doctors warned that they would lead to an epidemic of unhealthy posture.

lounge compressed the internal organs and could lead to a host of health problems, from indigestion to infertility.

This was a real worry at the time, but as you can see from the photos, those lounges were pretty mild by today's standards. We'll talk more about the bizarre history of American posture later in this book, but for now I'm going to need to break a bit of bad news: your couch is bad for you.

Don't worry, I'm not about to suggest diligently sitting ramrod straight as you binge watch TV deep into the night. But I do have a few tweaks that'll help you keep your couch from foiling your posture progress.

Simply throwing a few pillows under your lower back can go a long way toward keeping your posture from collapsing. Think about lengthening your spine whenever you're sitting on your couch. It doesn't take any effort, just the strategic placement of a few throw pillows. Even if your back is a little rounded in this position, at least all of your bodyweight is being supported. The worst problems come when your rounded spine is being relentlessly pushed into that position by the weight of your entire body.

Better yet, lie on the couch instead of sitting on it. Or, best of all, lie on the floor. Simply lying on the floor with a small pillow under your head is training your spine to lengthen and relax. Think about letting your body sink into the floor under the weight of your bones. Let gravity do all the work. *Voila*! Great posture without any effort.

I know, I know, you still love your couch. Believe it or not, as your posture improves you'll soon start to feel uncomfortable sitting on most couches. Just in case avoiding physical pain isn't enough of a reason to ditch your couch, you might want to consider the possibility that healthy posture can make you less anxious and depressed, more confident, and even more successful. It's true! And that's the topic of our next chapter.

8

NEW POSTURE, NEW YOU

I was once interviewed on a television show where I had to sit on a particularly soft couch with a very deep seat, which seemed ironic because I was there to talk about the benefits of healthy posture. When I saw it, I immediately felt a jolt of anxiety. How could I look authoritative while fighting to keep the enormous couch from swallowing me up? I wanted my body language to project confidence, but that seat was designed to push my body into a terrible slump.

When I'm sitting tall, I know that I look confident, which makes me feel confident. And when I'm helplessly molded into the shape of my chair, I feel self-conscious and socially awkward.

Just when I was on the brink of panic, I took a deep breath and thought about "The Big Three." I perched myself on the edge of the couch, not daring to let my bottom venture into the back half of the seat. With my sitz bones anchored and my upper body open and relaxed, I could gesture freely and breathe deeply. As a result, my voice came out sounding strong and confident, and my body was poised and comfortable.

Even though I was nervous about being on live television, I looked (and felt) comfortable in my own skin.

Fake It Till You Make It

Stanford Graduate School of Business is one of the top business schools in the world. Located in the heart of Silicon Valley, it's a sort of incubator for the cutting-edge innovators of tomorrow. Students pay big bucks to get access to the secrets of success.

A popular class there is called Acting with Power. It teaches MBA students how to project confidence, and it's co-taught by a professor from the drama department! Who better than an actor to analyze the subtle emotional messages that can be conveyed through body language?

The course description says the class, "is designed specifi-cally for students who have trouble 'playing' authoritative roles: those who find it difficult to act with power, status, and authority."

The class sounds amazing, but just in case you don't have tens of thousands of dollars and a Stanford-worthy GPA, I know another way to project a calm authoritative presence. The answer, of course, is to stop acting and start being. It's actually much easier than it sounds.

There's new research showing that healthy posture can make you feel more assertive and less stress reactive. In other words, your posture doesn't just make you look confident, it creates the feeling of confidence too!

Be A Power Poser

Have you ever watched a submissive dog meet a dominant one? He makes himself small, bowing his head and rounding his whole spine. You'll recognize it as a posture that's universal throughout the animal kingdom. Dominant animals take up space and move with relaxation, while submissive ones make themselves small and tense.

Dominant and submissive animals hold themselves differently, and they behave differently. We now know that they

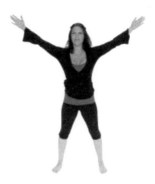

Open posture can make you feel powerful and confident.

also think differently. This is interesting, since most people spend their days hunched in front of screens with the body language of a submissive animal.

When scientists measured the hormones in dominant and submissive chimpanzees, they found that the two groups have dramatically different brain chemistry. The dominant chimps have higher levels of testosterone (the dominance hormone) and lower levels of cortisol (the stress hormone).

Amy Cuddy, a researcher at Harvard Business School, gave a popular TED Talk on this very subject. She says that it's possible to alter the levels of these hormones in humans, simply by asking them to hold their bodies a certain way. When people held expansive, powerful positions for just two minutes, their testosterone levels rose and cortisol levels dropped, said Cuddy. The results were exactly the opposite for those who held small, meek positions.

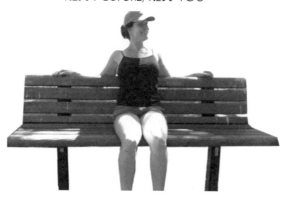

Not only is this confident posture, it's a great chest stretch!

Why are business schools interested in such a thing? Because it gives you a competitive edge. Cuddy sent people into mock interview situations and found exactly what she'd expected – those who had held a "power pose" for just two minutes prior to the interview performed much better, according to a panel of neutral judges who didn't know if the subject had held a powerful pose or not.

I thought about this research before my last job interview. I stood in the parking lot with my arms outstretched and my torso long just before going in. I was a little worried that people would see me standing there and wonder if I was crazy, but otherwise it felt really good! Even if it didn't improve my performance, it did give my muscles a nice stretch, which left me feeling more relaxed.

If something as simple as holding a pose for two minutes can alter your brain chemistry to give you a competitive advantage, just imagine what a lifetime of healthy posture can do.

Boob-Shaming and Women's Posture

The very first time I remember being boob-shamed I was 15-years old. I was wearing a white t-shirt and jeans at an outdoor concert and I forgot to bring a sweater. When the sun went down it started to get cold. As I stood there shivering, a random guy came up to me, looked at my chest and said, " Your headlights are on." His friends thought it was hilarious.

Unfortunately, most women have at least one story about a time when they were made to feel ashamed of their breasts. Just last week, a friend told me a story about a boob-shaming experience that she had at work. She's a highly educated scientist in a senior position at her company. She was bending over a workbench, working on something that caused her to hold her arms in close to her body. Even though she was wearing a modest shirt that barely dipped below her collarbone, there was a little cleavage showing. A male colleague complained that it was distracting and HR ended up getting involved – not to discipline the man, but to discuss her boobs before finally deciding that her shirt was okay to wear at work after all.

We're taught that it's not polite to have big breasts. People find them distracting, cheap or disgusting (just try breastfeeding in public). Some of the worst posture problems that I've seen belong to women with large chests who collapse downward to avoid unwanted attention.

It's no wonder that many women often struggle to improve their posture. If you're used to sinking your chest down, it might feel like you're showing off a bit once you start to change. My friend's mom used to always ask her, "Why do you always flaunt your chest like that?" She was a professional dancer with healthy posture and a large bra size, but she wasn't flaunting anything. She was simply holding her chest in a healthy, neutral position, but even her own mother seemed to find it offensive.

Society teaches women to take up as little space as possible, so we round our shoulders, cross our legs and waste a lot of energy making our bodies small. I hadn't thought about it that much until hearing a lecture in a sociology class, but women also yield the right of way to men on busy sidewalks, shy away from shared armrests, and tolerate "manspreading" on public transportation (when a man sits with his leg so far apart that he's taking up half the leg room of the person next to him).

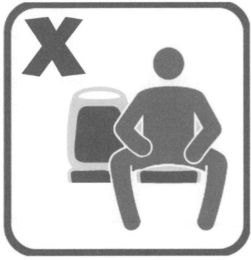

This "no manspreading" sign can be seen on public buses in Madrid, Spain. Men generally feel more free to take up physical space.

In order to change your posture, you first need to learn to be confident about taking up space. For most women, this is easier said than done.

The 10-Pound Rule

You've probably heard that old saying that the camera adds 10 pounds. But did you know that standing up straight instantly drops 10 pounds? When the front of your body is collapsed forward, your stomach has nowhere to go but out. Lengthening your torso has the same effect as sucking in your stomach, but it's way less effort!

I'm sure you've noticed that some people seem to wear their weight much better than others. I've noticed this with dancers time and time again. I once knew a dancer who was 20 pounds heavier than I was, but I didn't realize it until I wanted to buy one of her old costumes. I couldn't tell that she was several sizes larger than me, even when I was looking directly at her! It's no coincidence that she always had a regal and poised demeanor. She had a certain majestic quality about her that I couldn't put my finger on at the time. Of course, now I know her secret!

It's not just that healthy posture pulls in your stomach, it also makes you taller, redistributing many of the bulges that people tend to want to get rid of. Even the skinniest of people can produce rolls of fat by letting their posture collapse. So when you stand tall, you can feel confident that you're looking your very best!

Saving Grace

If you consider yourself to be an uncoordinated klutz, chances are that improving your posture will help with that too. Elite athletes will make the most difficult tasks look effortless, because they understand the importance of relaxing into their movement. By using only the muscles essential to the movements, an athlete keeps the rest of their body alert and without tension.

Has anyone ever told you that you're "trying too hard" when attempting a physical feat? That has to be the single most frustrating piece of advice that a beginner can receive! But it simply means that you're holding too much tension in places that should be relaxed. Tension draws your energy away from the intended movement. And what's the best way to get rid of muscle tension? Healthy posture!

9

POSTURE STRETCHES

I used to wear one of those step-counting devices, and I'd feel a sense of accomplishment whenever I reached 10,000 steps in one day. I'd park my car at the far end of the parking lot when I went grocery shopping, and take my dog for extra long walks in hopes of increasing my step count. After all, walking is good for you...right?

In addition to walking, I went to boot camp exercise classes several times a week. At the time, I didn't understand that all that exercise was only reinforcing my patterns of tightness. It's not that exercise is bad, quite the opposite, but the way I was exercising was bad for me!

I now know that in order to balance out my body and undo the effects of chronic sitting, I needed to stretch the front of my body and strengthen the back. All those push-ups and lunges at boot camp were tightening muscles that were already chronically tight. Even the way I walked was making all of the imbalances in my body worse.

When you have unhealthy posture, you're tensing muscles that you should be relaxing instead. In turn, when you exercise with bad form, you're further tightening up the muscles that pull you into unhealthy posture. I always ask gym rats to back off their workout for a few weeks while they're starting to change their posture.

Then, when they do return to the gym, they'll have better form and get more benefit from their workout. Plus, they'll use their knowledge of posture to rethink their whole workout routine. So many people do a disproportionate number of exercises that further tighten the tightest muscles (like those in the chest) and ignore muscles that are chronically weak due to unhealthy posture (like the ones in the upper back).

Pushups, sit ups, curls and lunges all target muscles that are already chronically tight in most people. All the muscles of the chest, the biceps and the quads are constantly shortened in modern life. We want to encourage them to lengthen and relax. In other words, they should be stretched, not tightened.

Tight Muscles Are Weak Muscles

Here's another reason why strengthening tight muscles is a bad idea: the tightness prevents them from being truly strong. I used to have rock-hard thigh muscles, which was something I was very proud of. I thought it was because I worked out, but when my back pain got really bad, I stopped exercising for a long time. Many other muscles became soft with neglect, but my thighs remained hard as rocks. And the strange part is that they would become tired and shaky whenever I walked uphill or got up from a squatting position.

I couldn't understand it. At least, not until I went to a physical therapist who told me that those muscles were full of adhesions. In other words, they were stuck, and scar tissue was cementing them in that position. In my case, it was most likely from overuse, but you can get muscle adhesion and knots as a result of an injury, or even from dehydration. The process of releasing that adhesion was not a pleasant one - a massage therapist had to basically dig in and rip it apart.

In the end, my thighs felt a lot softer, but they were a lot stronger as well. I now realize that the tightness in my thighs had prevented me from accessing the full strength of those muscles.

The moral of the story is that tight muscles are weak muscles. In order to strengthen them, you must first get them to relax. That's why you should always stretch as part of your workout. When your blood is pumping and your body is warm, that's the best time to stretch for the maximum results.

So many people neglect stretching, but if you're in the process of changing your posture, it's the single most important part of your workout. If you don't have time to do much, at least take 60 seconds to stretch out your chest.

The following pages are full of targeted stretches and exercises that are specifically designed to accelerate your posture progress! For maximum results do a few every single day.

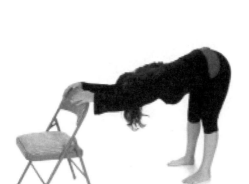

Chair Underarm Opener

Place your hands on the back of a chair and open your underarms, letting your body weight do all the work.

If the back of your legs are too tight to let you comfortably do this, simply bend your knees.

You can also try this on a higher surface like a kitchen counter.

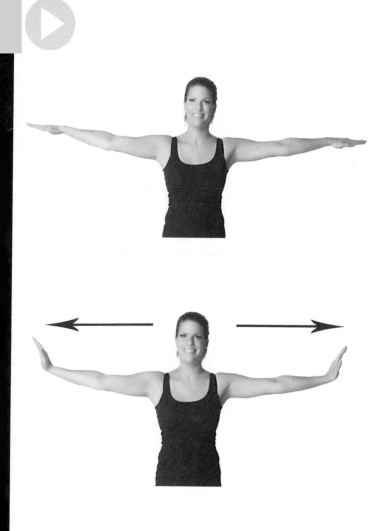

Straight Arm Push Away

Hold your arms out, shoulders relaxed and neck long. Take a deep breath. As you exhale, lift your fingertips toward the sky and push your palms away from each other. You should feel a stretch in your hands, arms and chest.

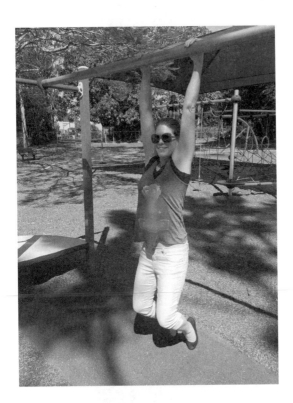

Hanging

Next time you see a chin-up bar, grab onto it and gently hang. This is an excellent shoulder stretch that also gives your back a bit of traction. You might even want to think about getting a home chin-up bar. There are several inexpensive models that can easily attach to a door frame.

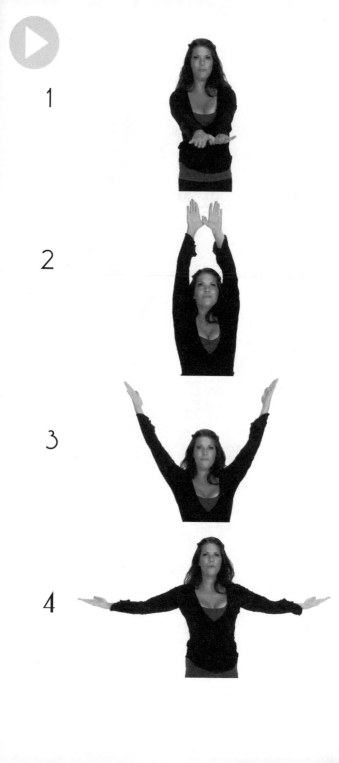

Reach Up, Reach Back

This is my favorite exercise of all time. I suggest doing 20 reps every single day. First, hook your thumbs in front of you (1). Then engage your upper back by pulling your arms away from each other so that if your thumbs weren't hooked your hands would fly apart.

While continuing to pull against your thumbs, raise your arms over your head (2). Keep your arms as straight as possible.

Then gently unhook your thumbs and let your palms face each other (3). Slowly lower your straight arms down (4). While lowering, pull your shoulder blades together in order to open your chest. This should be a nice stretch for the arms, chest and shoulders.

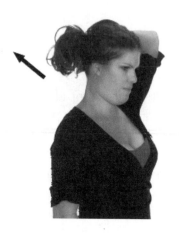

Diagonal Hair Pull

This simple stretch helps guide your head into the correct position. Grab a handful of hair at the base of your neck and gently pull it diagonally as you let your chin drop.

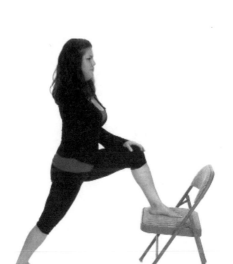

Chair Lunge

This is good for stretching out the hip muscles that get tight from chronic sitting. Just put your foot up on a chair and lean forward into a well balanced lunge. Be sure your back toes are facing forward and that your hip bones are parallel (people tend to let the hip bone on the straight leg side drift back).

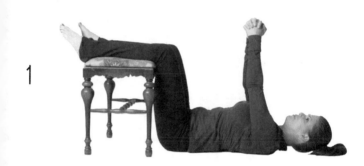

1

2

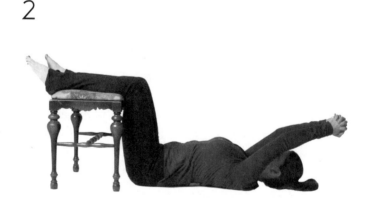

Overhead Floor Touch

I like to do this one with my legs up on a chair as seen in the photos, but it isn't necessary. Interlace your fingers and hold your arms out in front of you (1). While keeping your elbows as straight as you can, lift your arms over your head (2). Ideally, you will be able to touch your arms to the ground while keeping straight elbows.

I also like to use this position to do some active relaxation (seen below). It feels nice to let gravity straighten out your spine. I keep my palms up and think about opening my shoulders while breathing deeply.

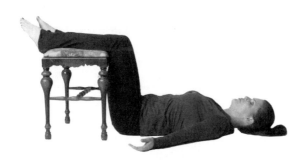

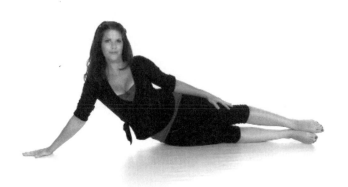

Lateral Line Floor Stretch

This stretch creates length in the torso. Be sure to avoid sticking out your bottom. You want your body to be in a perfectly straight line. If you have difficulty balancing, go ahead and place your top hand on the ground in front of you (be sure to avoid folding at the hips).

If the stretch in the photo is too deep, place your elbow on the ground instead of your hand. Breathe deeply and think about your side gently opening and melting toward the ground.

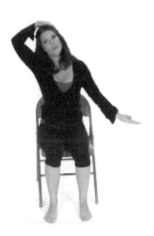

Straight Arm Neck Stretch

This opens all those tight muscles in your neck, shoulder and arm. With a straight arm (palm up) and a relaxed shoulder, gently tilt your head to the opposing side. Don't let that palm rotate forward, and be sure to keep your shoulder down.

For a deeper stretch you can place your hand on your head, like in the photo. But don't pull on your head. Simply let the weight of your arm give you an extra stretch. You should always be very gentle with your neck, so be sure to take this one slow.

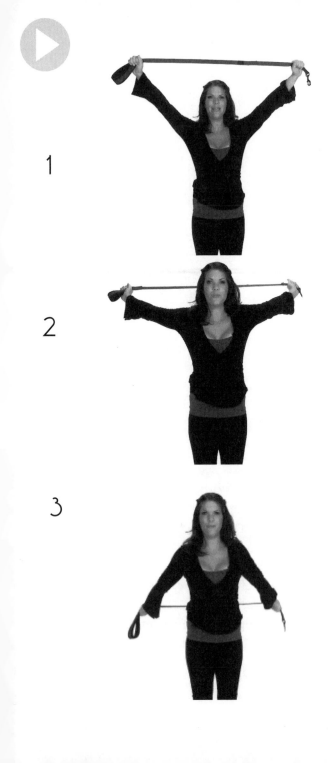

1

2

3

Towel Reach Over

I like to do this one with a towel just after taking a shower. In this demo, I'm using a dog leash, but you can use anything that's handy. Something that has a slight stretch (like an old pair of sweatpants) will make it less challenging.

Start off with your hands very far apart. Reach over your head (1) then down the back of your body (2 & 3). The key is to keep your elbows straight the whole time. The wider you hold the towel, the easier it will be. Over time you can move your hands closer together.

You can also turn this into a side stretch by leaning to the side with your towel overhead (seen below).

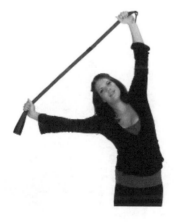

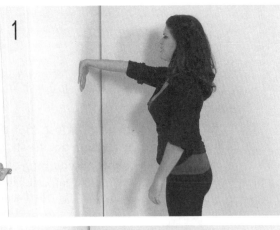

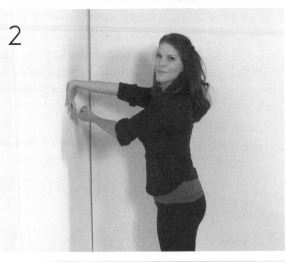

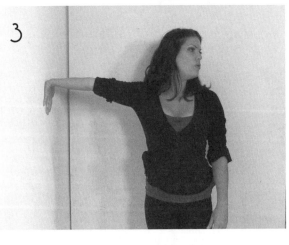

Wall Twist Away

This stretch opens your hands, arms, shoulders and neck. First, place your palm flat against a wall with your fingers pointing down (1). For some, this will be enough of a stretch.

If you'd like an additional forearm stretch, gently pull one finger at a time away from the wall (2 & below).

Then rotate your body away from the wall to move the stretch into your whole arm (3). If you'd like more, turn your head and look away from your hand.

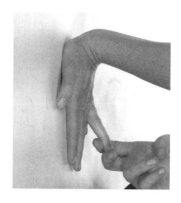

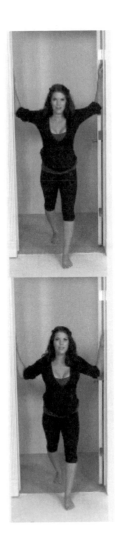

Doorway Stretch

Place your hands and elbows on a door frame and lunge forward until you feel a chest stretch. Be sure to repeat this stretch a few times with your arms in slightly different positions.

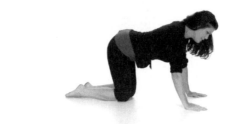

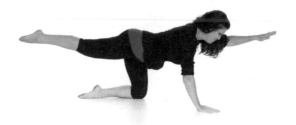

The Flag

While on your hands and knees, slowly extend the opposite arm and leg. Hold for 20-30 seconds. This will build muscle in the whole back side of your body.

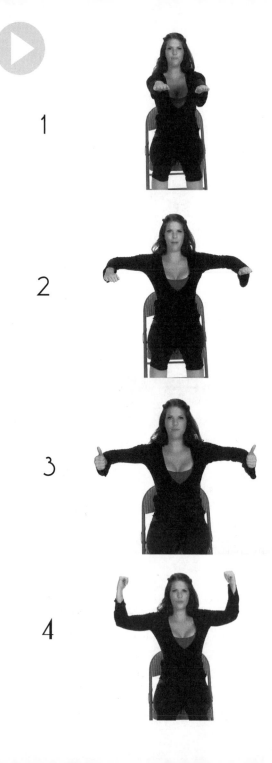

Seated Rows

This back strengthening exercise can be done sitting or standing.

Start with your arms outstretched in front of you (1) then pull your elbows back as far as you can (2). Be sure your armpits and elbows are at right angles.

Then rotate your hands and do a thumbs up (3). Rotate your arms upward and point your thumbs behind you (4).

I prefer to do this exercise with my back against a wall so that my elbows and thumbs have a target to hit. It keeps me honest!

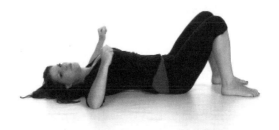

Elbow Push Back

This is a great way to build muscle in your upper back!
Place your elbows on the ground with fists toward the
ceiling. Make sure that your armpits and elbows are at
right angles. Now push your elbows into the ground as
hard as you can.

Hold this for 20-30 seconds. Even though your position
won't change, you should be using a lot of energy to do
this exercise.

10

ΛFTERWORD

We've covered a lot of information in this book, but the truth is that transforming your posture is not that complicated. Just remember, everything revolves around "The Big Three." If your sitz bones are anchored, your chest is open and your neck is long, you're well on your way! New habits will start to develop and your body will start to change for the better.

Just the act of thinking about your posture will help you transform the way your body moves and feels. You don't have to set an alarm to remind yourself to sit up straight, because looking at other people will remind you every day. You won't be able to help noticing the epidemic of unhealthy posture everywhere you go, and you also won't be able to help wincing in empathy.

As you start to feel better, it will become addictive. Maybe you'll even find yourself absentmindedly stretching your chest by resting your arm behind the passenger's seat as you drive. Or maybe you'll fling your arms over the backrest next time you're sitting on a park bench. As your body starts to crave open, relaxed posture, it will become easier and easier to maintain.

And if you're still having trouble getting relief from the tension that unhealthy posture has created, it probably just means that you need to stretch. If you would prefer to learn from a video, I demonstrate all of these stretches (and many more) on my website www.posturemakeover.com (the password for the Book Club page is Postur3).

Your initial transition into healthy posture is the hardest part. Once you get over the fact that it feels weird and that it requires a lot of brainpower to change your habits, you'll feel a deep sense of satisfaction at your incredible transformation.

As you settle into your new posture, you'll start to grow into a whole new you. You'll feel more light and open, confident and coordinated. When you're visibly comfortable in your own skin, you'll radiate a sense of well-being and satisfaction. And when people ask, "What's your secret?" Just tell them you've had a posture makeover!

FORGOTTEN LESSONS

One of my favorite parts about researching this book was discovering the fascinating history of American posture. I couldn't resist telling you all about it.

The most frustrating thing about seeing so many young people with such unhealthy posture is knowing that America used to be a nation obsessed with the posture of our children! Posture was a mandatory subject in schools all the way up through the college level. And it wasn't an arbitrary decision. It happened because of a massive public outcry, heated political debate, and a well-organized social movement.

It's part of a forgotten chapter that I rediscovered while poring over obscure academic journals deep in the Stanford University library. I had no idea that there was once a large-scale social movement to protect the posture of children! Looking back, some of their beliefs seem outdated, bizarre

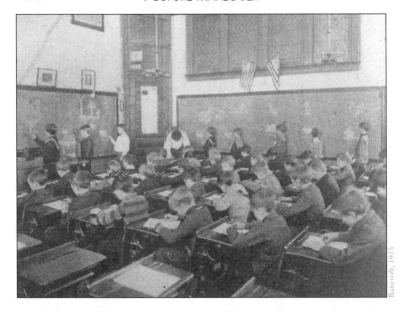

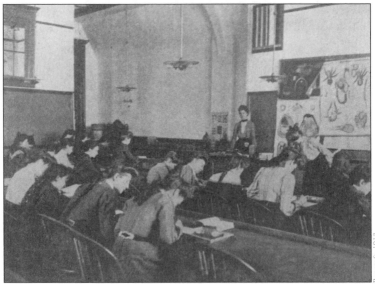

Many parents were horrified at the thought of their children spending the whole day sitting in a chair.

or just plain wrong (for example, they thought that bad posture led to immoral behavior). And in the end, their ideas were relegated to the dustbin of history. But in many ways, they were ahead of their time. There's plenty of forgotten wisdom in their teachings, if we care to look.

"Don't Make Our Kids Sit All Day!"

It all started with an idea that doesn't seem so controversial today – compulsory schooling for all children. But back in the late 1800s, this was a radical concept.

Children usually worked in the family business from a young age. Then the government said they should all go to school instead.

To make matters worse, children would have to spend six hours a day stuck behind a desk. Horrified parents argued that growing bodies needed freedom and exercise, and that all that time spent sitting down would make their children weak and sickly.

This hot-button political issue was even featured in the Democratic Party's national platform in 1892: "We are opposed to state interference with parental rights and rights of conscience in the education of children."

Faced with a growing insurrection, the school system needed a way to de-escalate the situation. So they vowed that they'd protect the health of their students, doing everything possible to keep them safe from the harmful effects of chronic sitting. With the future of public education resting in the balance, they turned to an unlikely savior – The American Posture League.

Mandatory Posture Classes

Just as the controversy was reaching fever pitch in 1913, The American Posture League was born. Its task: to make sure every last child in the public school system had pristine posture. No one questioned why this was an important undertaking.

"In good posture, also, better circulation, respiration, and digestion keep the stores of energy and sense of well-being at a higher level, and the efficiency and even the spirits of the individual are thereby placed on a loftier plane," wrote Jessie Bancroft, one of the founders of the posture movement.

Posture evaluations became a regular part of school. Children who didn't pass the posture tests were separated from the class and assigned therapeutic stretches and exercises until their posture improved. PE classes were geared toward

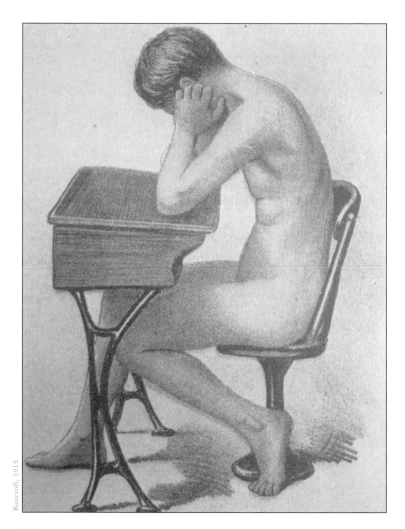

Volumes were written about the hazards of an ill-fitting desk.

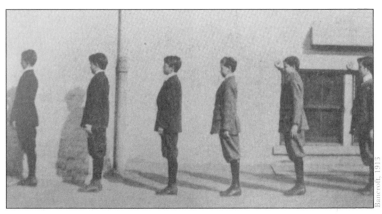

These boys all passed their weekly posture test.

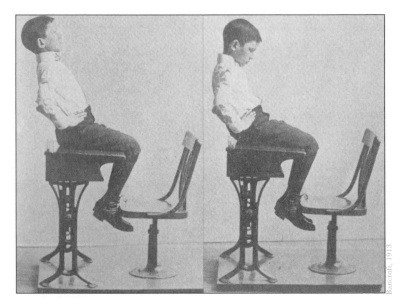

This photo demonstrates the right and wrong way to make children do situps at their desks.

posture correction (in fact, the founder of the modern PE movement, Dr Elisa Mosher, was also a co-founder of the American Posture League) and any posture problem was swiftly stomped out. Everything from a forward head to a pigeon toe was addressed, while the watchful eye of teachers made sure that bad habits never returned.

School furniture was ingeniously turned into exercise equipment, and teachers routinely made the classroom into a sort of makeshift gym. Interestingly, variations of their exercises are still prescribed by physical therapists today for patients with injuries resulting from chronic sitting. Many children were likely spared from a lifetime of chronic pain as a result.

School administrators thought that healthy posture was key to good health, and believed that unhealthy posture could lead to many different disabilities and diseases. Even after they understood the role that germs played in the spread of disease, it was still widely believed that collapsed posture could make you more susceptible to lung diseases like tuberculosis. The logic was straightforward: slumped posture puts pressure on the lungs, keeping them from functioning properly and making it difficult to fight off the disease.

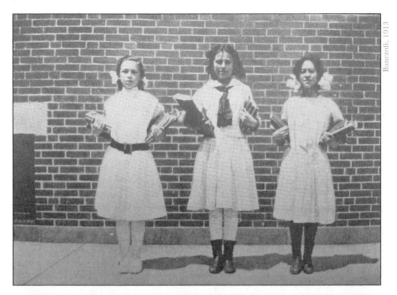

Bancroft, 1913

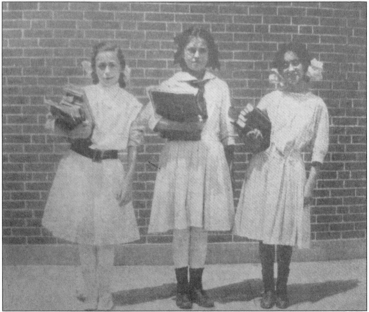

These girls are demonstrating the hazards of holding heavy schoolbooks on one side of the body. Distributing the weight evenly between both arms keeps the body balanced.

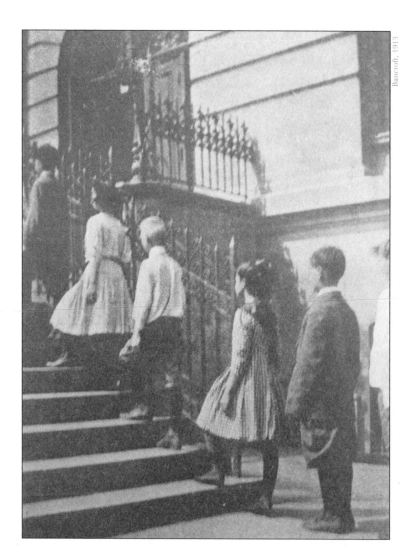

Bancroft, 1913

Part of the standardized posture test involved walking up stairs. Anyone who leaned forward automatically failed.

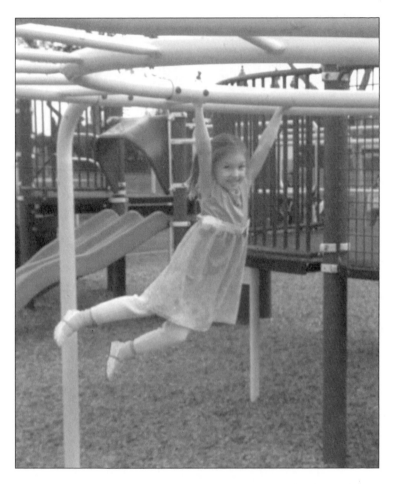

Monkey bars were invented in 1920 as a therapeutic tool to help children stretch out their chests, in hopes of protecting them from deadly infections.

The connection between healthy posture and breath was a large part of the curriculum, and it was not uncommon for teachers to ask students to gather around an open window and practice breathing deeply as part of their posture lesson. It wasn't just because they thought fresh air was nice, they literally felt that they were saving children's lives.

Ok, That's a Little Much

Sadly, the genius of the American Posture League was tainted with what would definitely be considered abuse in this day and age. Though the posture lessons and evaluations were revolutionary, the motivational techniques left a lot to be desired.

Not only did every child get graded on their own posture, but classrooms that didn't measure up received collective punishment. One PE teacher in Detroit was quoted as proudly saying, "in a particularly ambitious room the lives of the poor [children with bad posture] are made miserable until they straighten up."

Bancroft herself boasted that, "the boys in one class waylaid a classmate after school and pummeled him because his poor posture kept the class from one hundred per cent."

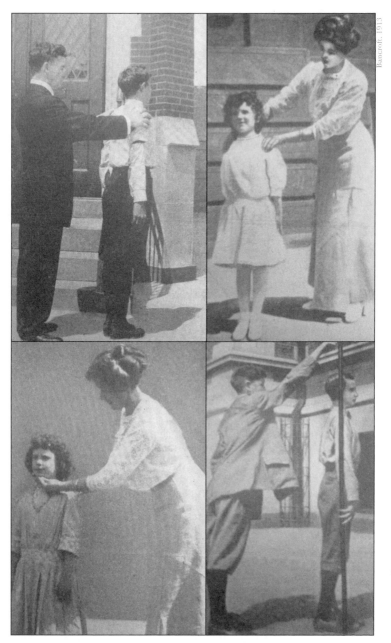

Bancroft, 1913

Teachers were trained in the art of posture evaluation and correction.

The image of innocent children being mercilessly beaten by their classmates just because they couldn't stand up straight is disturbing to say the least. And the fact that authority figures seem to have thought it was an appropriate motivational technique makes it even worse – a bit like finding out that "Lord of the Flies" happened during recess while the teachers were watching from the lounge.

Posture Police

If you think the elementary schools got carried away, you'll be shocked at what happened at the college level.

It is impossible to understate the enthusiasm of their posture crusade, especially at Vassar. Just in case you don't believe me, here's the class song from 1923: "When we get older / We won't be told ter / Keep a straight shoulder / It'll come natural / When you bend up like a bow / where do all your organs go / All of this you ought to know / She told us so."

The American Posture League insisted that body mechanics should be an ongoing, required course that was offered for credit at universities. They argued that only students of sound physical condition deserved a school's "full or highest diploma."

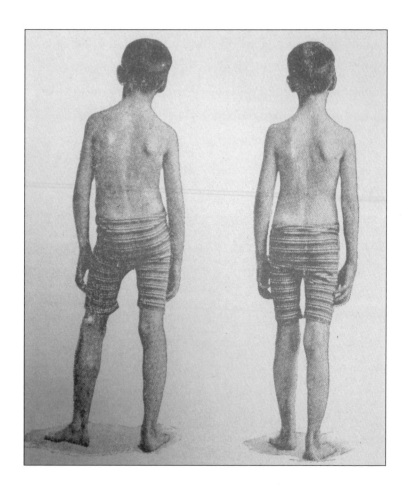

Instead of "hipping out" by throwing your weight to the side, The American Posture League suggested the position on the right instead.

Rigorous posture programs began appearing at elite universities in the 1920s, and continued to gain momentum throughout that decade.

Students who did not meet the standards of acceptable posture were routinely dismissed and denied their education! And if your posture was good enough to get you admitted, you were subjected to activities like Posture Day, where student "posture police" could walk around issuing tickets for posture infractions.

And you haven't even heard the worst of it yet!

The Naked Ivy League Posture Photo Scandal

I'd be remiss if I didn't mention a totally bizarre episode that involves prestigious universities taking naked posture pictures of their incoming freshmen. That's right, it was compulsory at many Ivy League schools to make students take mandatory nude photos.

This strange and disturbing trend emerged in the 1940s when universities such as Yale, Mount Holyoke, Vassar, Smith and Princeton began taking naked posture pictures of every incoming freshman. The photos were like a nude mug shot that recorded each student from the front, sides and back while in a standing position.

Reluctant students posed for nude photographs under the assurance that they were only to be used to track their posture progress, and would be destroyed upon completion of the course. But the photographs were not destroyed.

It was all very hush-hush until talk show host Dick Cavett made an off-color joke about it at a graduation ceremony in 1984.

"When I was an undergraduate...there were no women [at Yale]," Cavett told the audience. "The women went to Vassar. At Vassar they had nude photographs taken of women in gym class to check their posture. One year the photos were stolen and turned up for sale in New Haven's red-light district."

Then he delivered the punch line: "The photos found no buyers."

Feminist author Naomi Wolf, who was sitting in the crowd, didn't think it was funny. She told Cavett as much in a letter she wrote to The New York Times.

But the naked posture photos were still the stuff of legend until the 1990s, when The New York Times ran a story titled "The Great Ivy League Nude Posture Photo Scandal."

The most intriguing element was the surprising number of important public figures who were subjected to the practice. At Yale, George H.W. Bush, George Pataki and Bob Woodward were required to do it. Meryl Streep did it at Vassar. And Hillary Rodham and Diane Sawyer were photographed at Wellesley.

Newspaper columnist "Miss Manners" even weighed in on the proper etiquette for discovering naked posture photos of famous Ivy League women.

"There's a tremendous lesson here, which is that one should have sympathy and tolerance for respectable women from whose past naked pictures suddenly show up," she wrote.

Though the practice of nude freshman photos ended in the late 1960s, their bizarre legacy taints the modern view of the posture movement. A discussion about the commendable efforts of those who fought to improve the health and awareness of young adults inevitably devolves into the outrageous and creepy tale of teenagers being forced to disrobe for photographs.

"Proper" Posture, Sexism and Racism

Sadly, a look at the history of posture reveals other shocking examples of people going way too far. Beliefs about posture also got tangled up with the budding "science" of eugenics, the sexist and racist belief that physical traits influenced personality and intelligence. For example, Presidents Washington and Lincoln were said to have a classic physical trait of strong leaders: a long torso and short legs.

Back in the 1700s, erect posture and a long torso were seen as a signs of a proper, moral upbringing. If you were unlucky enough to have slumpy posture for any reason, people might think you had trouble controlling your lustful urges and a tendency toward deviant behavior in general.

Respectable people never slouched, partly because their clothing wouldn't allow it. Tight vests kept men's shoulders pulled back, while women (and even some men) wore corsets to keep their backs long and straight.

The Big Squeeze

Corsets had been around since the 15th century, but they really took off in the 1800s, thanks to the mass production that began during the industrial revolution. They became

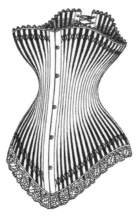

Drawing of a "luxury hourglass" corset from 1878.

all the rage because they flattened the stomach and created the illusion of full breasts – like an extreme version of Spanx combined with a pushup bra.

Corsets were also meant to help proper ladies maintain the proper posture. Mothers squeezed their young daughters into tight corsets in the hopes that they'd grow up with the kind of upright "ladylike" posture that'd make aristocratic gentlemen want to marry them. It was all very Jane Austen.

Even though the corset seemed to promote beautiful posture, it actually atrophied the core muscles due to lack of use. So, in a cultural climate where sitting up straight was supposed to be a sign of good character, women became too weak to do so without their corsets. It was a sort of crutch, or shortcut to create the illusion of a healthy body.

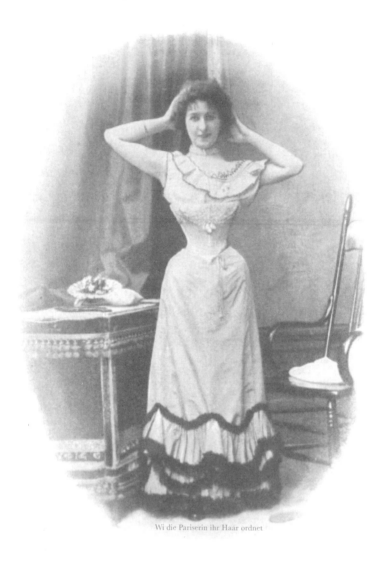

Wi die Pariserin ihr Haar ordnet

Tightly laced corsets were all the rage during the Victorian era.

Corsets had always been tight and uncomfortable, but it reached a whole new level during the Victorian era. Victorian women were obsessed with achieving an hourglass figure, and they used their corsets to squeeze their waists down to unbelievably small sizes. They called it "tight lacing."

If you could squeeze your waist down to 18 inches, you were doing well by the standards of the day – although many women achieved 16 inches or less. Just to give you a point of comparison, a healthy 130-pound woman today has a waist that's around 28-inches.

Dressed to Kill

It's no wonder women from this era suffered from dizziness and "fainting spells." Turns out that squeezing your lungs and other vital organs all day isn't the best idea.

Getting dressed was such an ordeal that some women ended up sleeping in their corsets without loosening them, just so they didn't have to do it all again the next morning. There were stories of mothers who pushed a foot into their daughters backs to gain an extra few inches, sometimes leading to broken laces, or even broken ribs. Plus, corsets were reinforced with whalebone stays, which sometimes broke and stabbed women through the stomach.

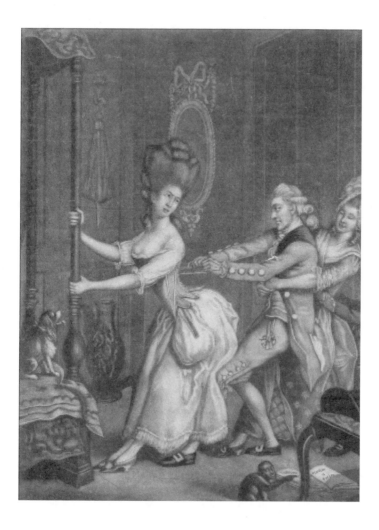

Every inch counts! Broken laces and broken ribs were not uncommon side effects of being squeezed into a corset. Some women slept in their corsets to avoid going through this painful morning ritual.

(Tight Lacing or *Fashion Before Ease, 1770)*

To make matters worse, corsets were often paired with a crinoline – a metal cage worn under a skirt in order to make it more puffy. These giant, flammable skirts often ended up brushing against candles and lanterns and catching on fire. A burning skirt on top of a crinoline was nearly impossible to put out, since the metal frame gave the fire plenty of air while making it impossible to roll on the ground to extinguish the flames. When a snarky observer coined the phrase "dressed to kill," they meant it literally.

Eventually, a movement emerged that recognized the damage that corsets were doing to women's health. "Anti-fashion" activist Luke Limner wrote in 1874 that corset-wearers were setting themselves up for a "sickly and short life."

He linked tight corsets to no less than 97 diseases, running the gamut from mental and reproductive, to digestive and cardiovascular ailments. He even blamed ugliness in children on their corset-wearing mothers. (Taking everything a step too far seems to have been a hallmark of the Victorian era).

Limner also recognized the link between an active rural lifestyle and better posture (which we covered in Chapter 5), although he described it in cringe-worthy terms, writing that the "inferior provincial classes and peasantry" in Europe were "undeformed."

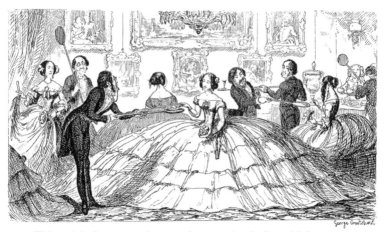

This satirical cartoon shows waiters serving ladies with long-armed trays, so that they can reach past their oversized skirts.

(The Comic Almanack, 1850)

Facing a growing backlash, corset makers tried marketing a new "healthful" version that was slightly less stiff. Various new corsets were introduced at the beginning of the 20th century, most of them claiming to be healthier than previous models. But as a national awareness about the benefits of exercise swelled, women started buying increasingly flexible clothing that facilitated free movement, and corsets became flimsier, with most women abandoning them altogether by the 1920s.

Slouching Becomes Cool

When women finally decided they'd had enough of the corset, it was a bold and radical gesture. These pioneering women were in a way even more radical than their bra-burning great granddaughters in the 1970s.

It's no wonder the flappers in the 1920s thought it was cool to slouch. It was an act of rebellion and feminism. It showed their affiliation with the counterculture. It shirked the repressiveness of the Victorian era. Slouching became a hallmark of a forward-thinking new generation. Of sexual liberation. Of modernity.

Slouching is still cool. Just look at any magazine or album cover. Many people are so used to seeing slumped posture that they now think it's completely normal. Even though the details of posture throughout history have been forgotten, the aftertaste remains. "Good" posture is still associated with Victorian era prudishness and upper class snobbery.

Back To The Future

But I think that's all starting to change. The rise of posture monitoring gadgets and ergonomic gizmos shows that posture is reemerging in our collective consciousness. People are beginning to think about the connection between posture and health again.

Though unhealthy posture had to reach epidemic levels for us to arrive at this point, I think we're at the dawn of a new posture era. Our world of desk jobs and hand held devices has shone a spotlight on the reality that we are misusing our bodies.

People have understood the connection between posture and chronic pain for a long time. We don't need to reinvent the wheel. I think we are due for a new posture movement, taking lessons from the past and adding a modern twist. And I hope that you will be part of that change.

SMARTPHONE APP

30 Day Posture Makeover
Access 3 hours of video, showing over 100 posture tips,
tricks and stretches. Available for iPhone or Android.

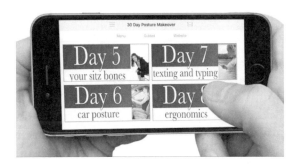

CHILDREN'S BOOK

Posture Posey and the Slumpyback Goblins
Instead of nagging your child to sit up straight (which won't help
anyway), you can make them feel like a superhero as they chase
the Slumpyback Goblins away.

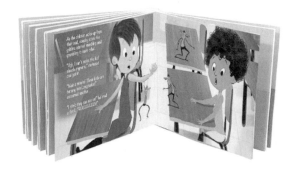

www.posturemakeover.com

BIBLIOGRAPHY

Allen, Frederick Lewis. *Only Yesterday, An Informal History of the 1920s*. Harper & Row, 1931.

Bancroft, Jessie H. *The Posture of School Children*. New York: The Macmillan Company, 1913.

Carney, D.; Cuddy, A. J. C.; & Yap, A. *"Power posing: Brief nonverbal displays affect neuroendocrine levels and risk tolerance."* Psychological Science, 21, 1363-1368 (2010).

Center for Disease Control and Prevention. "Musculoskeletal Disorders and Workplace Factors - A Critical Review of Epidemiologic Evidence for Work-Related Musculoskeletal Disorders of the Neck, Upper Extremity, and Low Back." Posted July 1997. https://www.cdc.gov/niosh/docs/97-141/default.html

Cuddy, Amy; Wilmuth, Caroline A; Yap, Andy J. and Carney, Dana R. *"Preparatory Power Posing Affects Nonverbal Presence and Job Interview Outcomes."* Journal of Applied Psychology 100, no. 4 (July 2015): 1286–1295.

Ethel Perrin. *"Methods of interesting school children in good postural habits."* American Physical Education Review, Vol 19 No 7 (Oct 1914).

Ewings, Elizabeth. *Dress and Undress: A history of Women's Underwear*. New York: Drama Book Specialists, 1978.

Harvard Health Blog. "Too much sitting linked to heart disease, diabetes, premature death." Posted January 22, 2015. http://www.health.harvard.edu/blog/much-sitting-linked-heart-disease-diabetes-premature-death-201501227618.

The Home School Court Report. "Compulsory Education Laws: The Dialogue Reopens." Posted October 2000. http://

nche.hslda.org/courtreport/v16n5/v16n501.asp

Hoy, Damian; Bain, Christopher; Williams, Gail; March, Lyn; Brooks, Peter; Blyth, Fiona; Woolf, Anthony; Vos, Theo and Buchbinder, Rachelle. *"A Systematic Review of the Global Prevalence of Low Back Pain."* Arthritis & Rheumatism, Vol. 64, No. 6 (June 2012): 2028–2037 DOI 10.1002/art.34347.

Kailb, Claudia. "The Great Back Pain Debate." *Newsweek.* May 2004. http://www.newsweek.com/great-back-pain-debate-127923

Kamitani, K; Michikawa, T; Iwasawa, S; Eto, N; Tanaka, T; Takebayashi, T; and Nishiwaki, Y. *"Spinal Posture in the Sagittal Plane Is Associated With Future Dependence in Activities of Daily Living: A Community-Based Cohort Study of Older Adults in Japan."* The Journals of Gerontology Series A: Biological Sciences and Medical Sciences (2013); DOI: 10.1093/gerona/gls253.

Kimiko. *Walking Your Way to a Better Life.* New York: Vertical, Inc., 2009.

Levine, James. *Get Up! Why Your Chair is Killing You and What You Can Do About It.* Palgrave MacMillan. 2014.

Limner, Luke. *Madre natura versus the Meloch of fashion, a social essay.* Oxford University, 1874.

Pheasant, Stephen. *Ergonomics, Work and Health.* Gaithersburg, Maryland: Aspen Publishers, Inc., 1991.

Pepper, Erik and Lin, I-Mei. *"Increase or Decrease Depression: How Body Postures Influence Your Energy Level."* Biofeedback Association for Applied Psychophysiology & Biofeedback, Volume 40, Issue 3, pp. 125–130 www.aapb.org DOI: 10.5298/1081-5937-40.3.01

Macdonald, Glynn. *Alexander Technique: A Practical Program for Health, Poise, and Fitness.* Element Books Limited, 1998.

Harland, Marion. *Eve's Daughters; or, Common Sense of the Maid, Wife and Mother*. New York: C. Scribner's Sons,1882.

Napheys, George. *Physical Life of Women*. Toronto: Maclear & Company, 1871.

Psych Central. "Poor Posture Can Affect Mood, Energy." Posted October 6, 2015. https://psychcentral.com/news/2012/10/16/poor-posture-can-affect-mood-energy/46112.html

San Francisco State University. "Research on posture yields insight into treating depression." Last updated January 29, 2016. http://news.sfsu.edu/research-posture-yields-insight-treating-depression.

Porter, Kathleen. *Natural Posture for Pain-Free Living*. Healing Arts Press, 2013.

Sawyer, Thea. *Put Your Back at Ease*. Live In Balance, 2013.

Schweizerischer Nationalfonds zur Foerderung der wissenschaftlichen Forschung. "Fear feeds the pain: Suffering from lumbago." *ScienceDaily*. www.sciencedaily.com/releases/2013/10/131017080104.htm.

Simplyhealth. "iPosture generation facing a lifetime of back pain." Posted October 2, 2013. http://newsroom.simplyhealth.co.uk/iposture-generation-facing-a-lifetime-of-back-pain/

Stearns, Peter N. *Battleground of Desire: The Struggle for Self-control in Modern America*. NYU Press, April 1, 1999.

Rosenbaum, Ron. "The Great Ivy League Nude Posture Photo Scandal." *New York Times*, January 15, 1995. http://www.nytimes.com/1995/01/15/magazine/the-great-ivy-league-nude-posture-photo-scandal.html.

Tyler, John Mason. *Growth and Education*. Houghton, Mifflin & Co., 1907.

Volinn, E. *"The epidemiology of low back pain in the rest of the world: A review of surveys in low-and middle-income countries."* Spine. (1997) 22(15):1747-54

Vassar College archives. "A memorandum on the need of a new physical education building at Vassar College." September 12, 1930.

Vallfors B. *"Acute, Subacute and Chronic Low Back Pain: Clinical Symptoms, Absenteeism and Working Environment."* Scandinavian journal of rehabilitation medicine. (1985) 11: 1-98.

Washington and Lee University. "Study links heavy texting, sleep problems in college freshmen." *ScienceDaily.* www.sciencedaily.com/releases/2013/09/130926111901.htm.

Waxman, Olivia B. "Study: Texting-While-Slouching Is Causing an 'iPosture' Epidemic." *TIME*. October 02, 2013. http://newsfeed.time.com/2013/10/02/study-texting-while-slouching-is-causing-an-iposture-epidemic/

White, Author and Kelly, Kate. *The Posture Prescription*. Three Rivers Press, 2001.

World Health Organization. *Priority Medicines for Europe and the World Update Report,* 2013. http://www.who.int/medicines/areas/priority_medicines/en/index.html.

Yosifon, David and Stearns, Peter N. *"The Rise and Fall of American Posture."* The American Historical Review, Vol 103, No. 4 (Oct., 1998) 1057-1095.